THE
MEDITERRANEAN
DIET
Made Easy

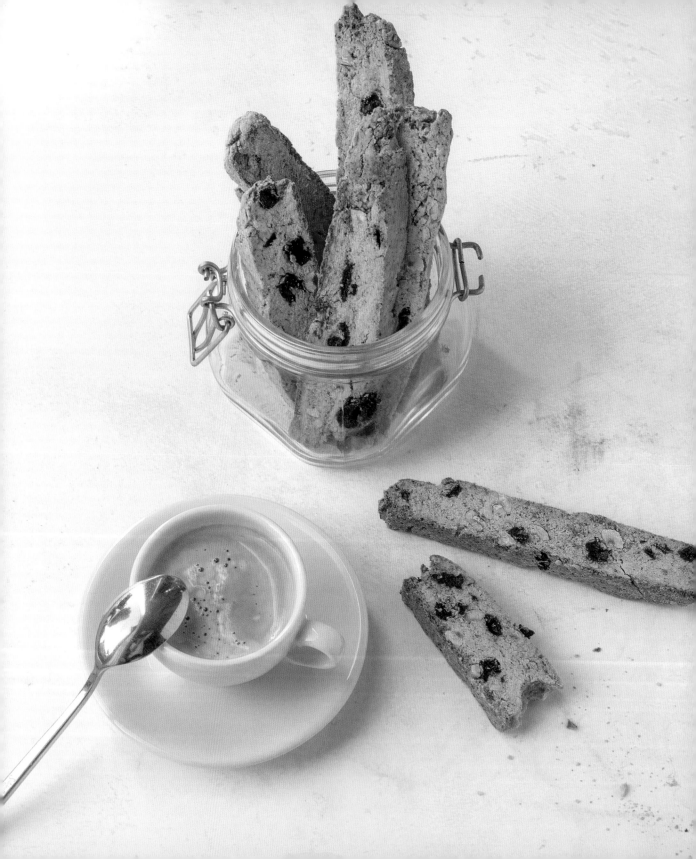

THE
MEDITERRANEAN
DIET
Made Easy

FRESH, VIBRANT RECIPES FOR
BETTER HEALTH

BRYNN MCDOWELL

CREATOR OF
THE DOMESTIC DIETITIAN

PAGE STREET
PUBLISHING CO.

Copyright © 2020 Brynn McDowell

First published in 2020 by

Page Street Publishing Co.

27 Congress Street, Suite 105

Salem, MA 01970

www.pagestreetpublishing.com

Distributed by Macmillan, sales in Canada by The Canadian Manda Group.

24   23   22   21   20   1   2   3   4   5

ISBN-13: 978-1-64567-074-2

ISBN-10: 1-64567-074-0

Library of Congress Control Number: 2019957231

Cover and book design by Rosie Stewart for Page Street Publishing Co.

Photography by Brynn McDowell

Printed and bound in China

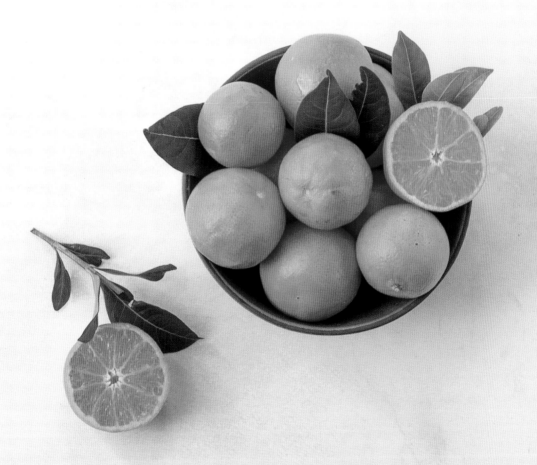

This book is dedicated to two very special people:

My husband, Dan, who has been my biggest supporter in every endeavor in my life.
You are always there to cheer me on and push me to step outside my comfort zone.
Your passion for everything in life is contagious. I love you.

My mom, Ruth, who passed on her never-ending love of cookbooks to me.
Thank you for always being there and teaching me about checking out
cookbooks from the local library.

Contents

HEALTHY SOUPS, SALADS AND SIDE DISHES

SIMPLE SWEETS AND TREATS

TIMESAVING SAUCES AND DRESSINGS

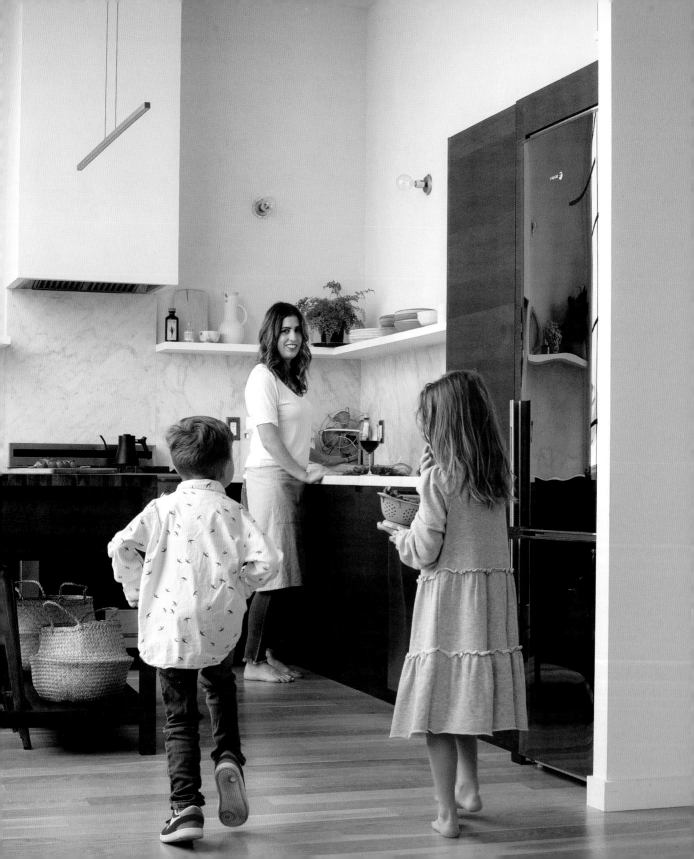

INTRODUCTION

Hi there! Chances are if you are reading this sentence then you've probably heard about the Mediterranean diet. Maybe you are curious about learning more about it, or you may be looking to make a change toward a healthier diet and need some help figuring out where to start. Or maybe someone gifted this book to you—in which case I suggest giving them a hug and making them a batch of the Almond and Cherry Baked Biscotti on page 156 as a thank-you.

All joking aside, whatever your reason is for picking up this book, I'm extremely happy that you did. Within these pages you'll discover why the Mediterranean diet has received the title of "best diet" multiple years in a row. It has also been named the best heart-healthy diet, best diet for diabetes management, best diet for healthy eating, best plant-based diet and easiest diet to follow.

The Mediterranean diet is one of the healthiest ways to live, and it's also realistic. It doesn't require special foods or forbid you from eating certain things. Instead, the focus is on real ingredients that can be found at the grocery store and some that are probably already in your fridge and pantry. It's completely customizable, so it's perfect if you are cooking meals just for yourself or if you are feeding your entire family. One of the things that first drew me to the Mediterranean diet is the emphasis on what to add to your meals rather than what to remove, something lacking in a lot of current diet recommendations.

I've always had a passion for things that involve health and nutrition. I can remember being about twelve years old and checking out a book from the library on becoming a vegetarian. I didn't want to become a vegetarian—mac and cheese with cut up hot dogs was just too good to even consider giving up at that point in my life—I just wanted to read and learn more about it. After changing my major four times in college, I stumbled upon a nutrition class and finally felt like I found something I could see myself doing forever. I graduated college with a degree in nutrition and food science, and then I went on to become a registered dietitian—and I have not regretted that decision once.

Still, I always thought I was missing something that tied together my views about nutrition and real-life balance in a way that I could explain and share with others. I didn't have a specific focus, such as diabetes management or sports nutrition. I had a general philosophy about health that involved eating fresh food as much as possible and limiting junk food—but not depriving yourself by eliminating entire food groups. I have always loved food and believe that the old adage "everything in moderation" applies to so much in life. This never really resonated too well with people that wanted my advice on a quick fix or a checklist of things they could eat to help them become "healthier."

Fast forward to 2011, when a trip abroad to various parts of France, Italy and Greece with my husband led me to my passion for all things Mediterranean. I absolutely fell in love with the food, the culture, the traditions and the ideals that people had about food and health. With the Mediterranean diet principles and lifestyle, I felt like I was finally able to connect all the dots between what I believed as a general food philosophy.

Ever since then I've shifted my focus, both professionally and personally, to learning more about the Mediterranean diet. In 2015, I started a blog called The Domestic Dietitian that was designed to share my knowledge and excitement about general nutrition and health with others. As my knowledge and passion grew, I narrowed down the focus of the blog toward sharing information specific to helping others create a Mediterranean diet in their own home. The Domestic Dietitian is now a website and company designed to be an expert on a realistic approach to the Mediterranean diet and lifestyle. In addition to adopting a Mediterranean diet in my own home, I currently create all the content for The Domestic Dietitian, which includes providing nutrition expertise for many print and online publications, as well as counseling others to help them incorporate this healthy lifestyle in their own homes.

My goal is for this book to help you learn to appreciate what fresh, simple ingredients can provide our bodies and how good they make us feel. I'm confident that you'll come to appreciate that the Mediterranean diet can be adapted to your goals—whether it be better health in general, a better relationship with food, learning how to create healthy meals in the kitchen, reducing your risk for cardiovascular disease, improving your family's health and everything in between. I want to eliminate all the confusion, quick fixes, deprivation and negative attitudes about food and just get back to loving a good meal. I hope you are encouraged to feel confident in the kitchen and find joy in creating a nourishing meal for your family and friends.

Some of the recipes in this book are influenced by the meals I've enjoyed while traveling, and many are my own take on traditional dishes designed with the realities of time, family and budget in mind. One of the things I love most about the Mediterranean diet is that it's based on guidelines rather than strict rules, and that means everyone can interpret those principles and work them into their own lives. Some of the recipes in this book aren't necessarily dishes you would find on a menu in Greece; instead they are designed to show that you can take any type of dish and make a few simple changes to put a Mediterranean spin on it. The focus is on using fresh, seasonal ingredients to create flavorful, nutritious, delicious meals that fit into your life.

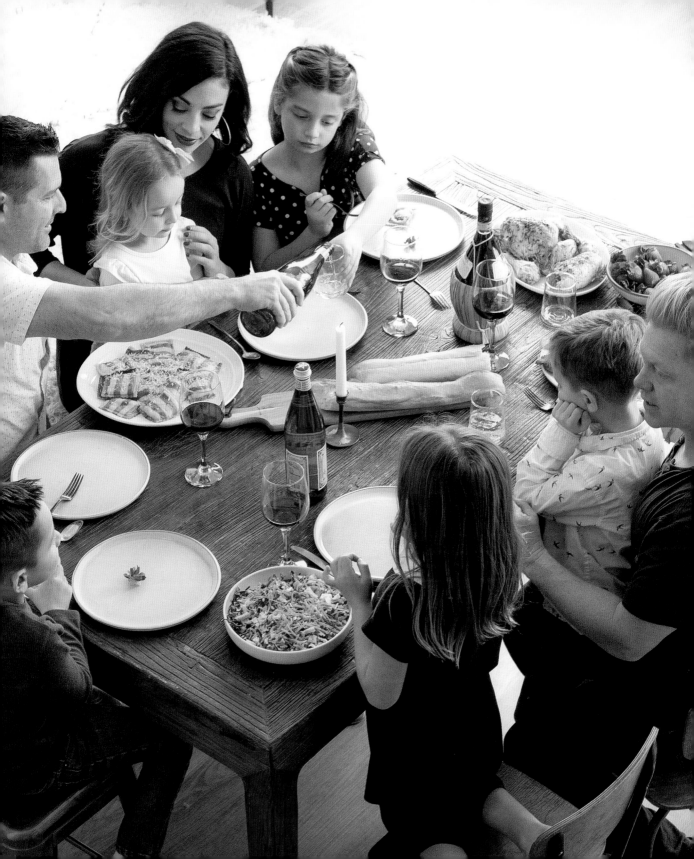

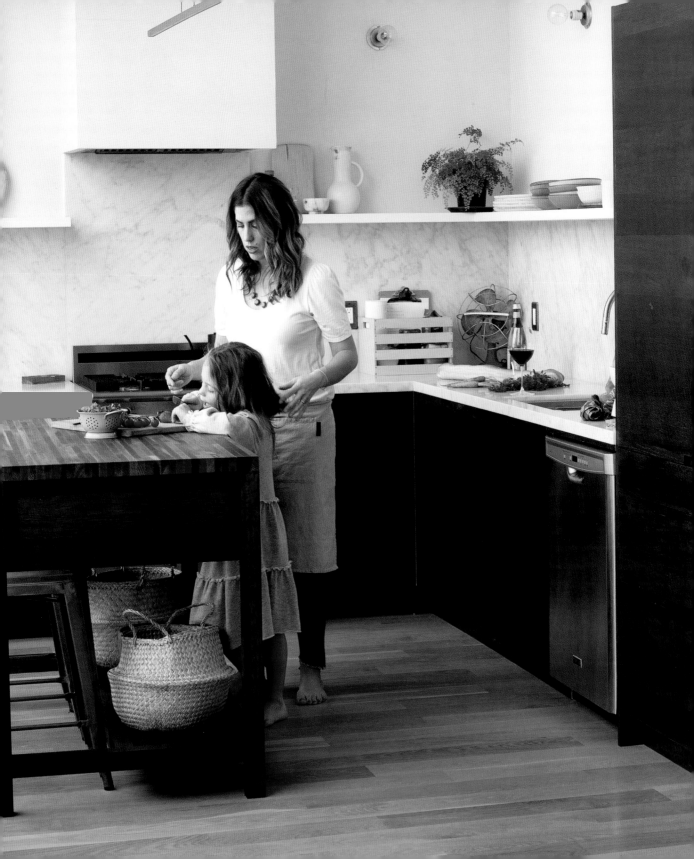

THE MEDITERRANEAN DIET: A WAY OF LIFE

We live in an age when people are looking for everything to be as fast as possible. The fastest Internet connection, quick replies via text, ten-second elevator pitches, the fastest route from point A to point B, fast food and ready-made meals. The Mediterranean diet is the complete opposite of our desire for a quick-paced life—and I find that so refreshing.

Rooted in centuries of tradition and culture, the Mediterranean diet is based on the eating patterns of the countries that border the Mediterranean Sea. Even though where we live no longer fully dictates what we eat, the guidelines of the diet can still be applied to create a healthy and happy lifestyle. In addition to the food, the Mediterranean diet puts an emphasis on physical activity, social connections and the joy that surrounds food. Health and nutrition are a balance of a lot of moving parts, and the Mediterranean diet truly looks at the bigger picture of wellness rather than one specific aspect of it.

The Mediterranean diet has been the focus of countless studies and analysis for decades. This is mainly because the people who follow this way of life have less incidence of chronic disease. Research has shown that following a Mediterranean diet may lead to reduced blood pressure, better control over blood sugars and lower cholesterol. The plant-focused diet offers a lot of anti-inflammatory and antioxidant-containing foods, which may help explain the possible reduced risk of stroke, heart disease, diabetes and cognitive decline—such as dementia and Alzheimer's—associated with this lifestyle.

THE MEDITERRANEAN DIET PRINCIPLES AND BENEFITS

Someone once asked me if they could still follow the Mediterranean diet if they didn't like olives. It was 100 percent a serious question. Of course my response was "yes," but it made me aware of just how strict we've become as a society about eating.

Unlike other diets that have very set rules and dictate what to eliminate from your meals, the Mediterranean diet is focused on what to add to your meals for health, nutrition and flavor. Nothing is off limits; instead it's more about finding the balance between foods eaten every day and those that are enjoyed as more of an occasional treat. The general guidelines suggest the following:

- **Daily:** fruits, vegetables, whole grains, legumes, nuts, seeds, olive oil, water
- **Often:** fish/seafood
- **Moderate:** poultry, eggs, cheese, yogurt, red wine
- **Occasional:** red meat, sweets

Daily

The heart of the Mediterranean diet focuses on building your meals around plenty of plant-based foods including fruits and vegetables, whole grains, legumes, nuts, seeds and olive oil. These foods contain nutrients that can help lower our risk for certain diseases or illnesses and provide us with protein, fiber and heart-healthy fats. Treating these foods as the star of our meals will help create balanced, nutrient-filled dishes that become the building blocks for many of the recipes in this book.

Often

The Mediterranean diet encourages incorporating seafood into meals a few times a week. Seafood contains essential omega-3 fatty acids that aren't created in high enough amounts in the body, so we have to obtain them from dietary sources. Research has shown that omega-3s can help promote healthy brain development in children and reduce the risk of heart disease in adults. Salmon, mackerel, tuna, herring and sardines have the highest amounts of omega-3s. The Monterey Bay Aquarium Seafood Watch website is a great resource if you are looking for more information on sustainable seafood choices.

Moderate

Poultry, eggs, cheese and yogurt are very much a part of the Mediterranean diet. They are encouraged in smaller portions, on a daily to weekly basis. While they aren't typically seen as the star of the show, there is certainly room for them. Often, they are used to finish off a dish or they are used as an accompaniment to the main dish. For example, you might serve a vegetable-filled salad with a sprinkling of feta cheese or top it with sliced grilled chicken.

There is still some debate about the type of dairy (fat free, low fat, full fat) that's recommended. On one hand, full-fat dairy is a source of saturated fat, which can increase cholesterol and risk for heart disease. On the other hand, some research indicates that full-fat dairy may decrease the risk for heart disease when compared to not eating dairy at all. In addition, dairy contains other nutrients—such as calcium, vitamin D and potassium—that may actually protect against some of the negative effects of saturated fat. My recommendation is to select the type of dairy you like best and enjoy it as part of a healthy lifestyle. I personally prefer full-fat dairy because I think it has a better consistency and more flavor, which actually means I am satisfied with a smaller amount of it.

Red wine is also recommended in moderation. Studies have shown that consumption of red wine can lead to a reduced risk of heart disease, but it's important to remember that better doesn't always mean more. I once had someone tell me that they don't like red wine, but they felt like they needed to start drinking it because of the health benefits. My response was that you shouldn't force yourself to eat or drink things you don't like for the sake of health, especially when it comes to alcohol. The key is moderation: one drink a day for women and two drinks a day for men. And it's important to remember that all alcohol, including wine, is associated with its own set of increased risks. If you don't currently drink alcohol or have certain medical conditions, it is not recommended that you start drinking just for the sake of it.

Occasional

Even though nothing is off limits, it is recommended that you consider red meat and sweets to be an occasional part of your lifestyle under the Mediterranean diet. They are still meant to be enjoyed—just less often than some other types of foods.

Red meat is typically higher in saturated fat. This can raise the levels of cholesterol in your blood, which can lead to an increased risk of heart disease and stroke. Choose a leaner cut of red meat, typically the ones with "round" or "loin" in the name. This is a simple change that can help lower saturated fat. However, it's also important to remember that nothing is "forbidden" in the Mediterranean diet. If you are enjoying red meat occasionally, as part of a balanced diet, then I say eat the cut that you enjoy and savor every bite.

The same can be said of sweets, especially those that are pre-packaged. Pastries, cookies and cakes can be heavy on empty calories, saturated fats and added sugars. They can still be enjoyed in moderation, but I recommend going for the real deal. By that I mean a homemade cake made with real sugar, chocolate, eggs, etc. Satisfy your cravings with real food rather than lackluster substitutes that aren't going to taste as great or leave you enjoying every bite.

It's also important to remember that this diet has been around for centuries and is considered one of the healthiest in the world because of the overall combination of foods. A single food or ingredient is not going to make or break your health. The Mediterranean diet isn't based on black-and-white rules. Even the above general guidelines are just that . . . guidelines. Everyone's life is different. Some days we may feel like we have it all together and on others it feels like nothing goes according to plan. Be flexible and allow yourself some grace.

LIVING A MEDITERRANEAN-INSPIRED LIFESTYLE

Health isn't made up of just the foods we eat, and I think the Mediterranean diet does a great job of reminding us of that.

One of my most memorable meals was a breakfast in Tuscany. In addition to the delicious dish that was prepared, the ease of the meal and the area where we enjoyed it really stood out to me. We sat in the morning sun at a table where the plates didn't match, no one was wearing shoes and everything was served family style. We sat next to complete strangers, but everyone came together and just enjoyed the meal and the conversation.

In moments like this I truly began to understand that a big part of the Mediterranean diet is the lifestyle that goes along with it. It is about taking the time to savor a meal, especially when shared with others. There is research that shows how enjoying a meal with another person can have an effect on our mood and mental health. I believe it also helps us slow down, keeping us from just eating as quickly as possible.

It's important to include the "non-food" elements of the Mediterranean diet. The following also play a big role in our overall health:

- Daily physical activity
- Plenty of sleep
- Stress management
- Nourishing your relationships
- Engaging in social connections

Of course we also have to live in the real world where there are schedules, meetings and life events that are out of our control. My advice is to truly figure out how this lifestyle can fit into your own day-to-day life. It will look different for everyone, but making the effort to include nutrition, physical health and mental health in your home will ultimately lead to a healthier you.

HOW TO START YOUR MEDITERRANEAN DIET

I'd say step number one to beginning your Mediterranean diet is reading this book—but I might be a little bit biased. All kidding aside, trying to change core areas of your lifestyle can be a bit overwhelming. The key to setting yourself up for success is making small changes. You have to find what works best for you and make it your own, one step at a time. Here are my tips to help get you started on your journey.

Slowly increase your intake of fruits and vegetables every day.

- Aim to include fresh fruits and/or veggies in every single meal. This can be as simple as adding vegetables to your pizza instead of pepperoni, or trying to incorporate fresh fruit in your dessert.
- Pick a vegetable that's new to you and find a new recipe to try. This will help you find new foods you like and new ways of preparing them.
- Try going meatless one night a week to incorporate more plant-based meals into your routine. Mushrooms, lentils and beans are great ingredients to add to meatless meals for hearty flavor.

Lean toward real ingredients.

- In general, the simpler a food is, the better. This is especially true when it comes to ingredients you've never heard of or can't pronounce such as additives, preservatives, coloring agents, thickeners, etc. Read the ingredients list on food labels and try choosing the products that are made with ingredients you recognize.
- If possible, try making more things at home instead of buying the heavily processed version. A great example is salad dressing: a vinaigrette takes a few ingredients and a few minutes to make, and you won't need the additives that are found in many store-bought versions.
- When a food is made with real ingredients, we are often more content with less. Choose real food rather than products designed to be low calorie or low fat.
- When food is flavored with fresh, natural ingredients, there is less need for heavy sauces, excess salt or added sugars. Avoid artificial flavors and sweeteners.

Stock your kitchen for success.

- Fresh ingredients are fantastic, but canned and frozen fruits and vegetables are also great—and much better than none at all.
- Dried beans and legumes make great pantry staples. They can be found at many stores in the bulk bins, so you only have to buy the amount you need. Just keep in mind that most of them require lengthy soaking before cooking. Timesaving tip: I rely on low-sodium canned beans and precooked lentils to pull together quick weeknight meals.
- Whole wheat pasta, brown rice, quinoa and barley can make great additions to meals. These grains also provide fiber, which is important for digestive health, and can improve cholesterol and blood sugar levels.
- Frozen fish, canned tuna and canned salmon can help you easily reach your goal of seafood twice a week.
- Stock your cabinet with plenty of flavor-enhancing herbs and spices such as dried thyme, basil, oregano, garlic, parsley, cumin, cinnamon, curry powder and red pepper flakes. Try new spice blends or create your own like the Greek Seasoning Spice Blend on page 177.

Get back to basics.

- Try cooking one more meal at home each week instead of going out to eat or buying pre-made items.
- Use what's in season. In-season fruit and vegetables often taste better and they're typically less expensive. Many of the recipes in this book indicate when the veggies listed can be swapped out for something else based on the season.
- Add more fresh herbs and spices to meals for flavor.
- If you aren't comfortable cooking, make it a goal to learn something new in the kitchen each week. It can be as simple as roasting vegetables or cooking chicken. The Internet is full of helpful videos. I used to have to look up how to make rice; we all start somewhere.

- If you are already at ease in the kitchen, try a new cooking technique. Grilling, braising, caramelizing and roasting can add a whole new dimension to even the simplest of ingredients.
- Remember, you don't need to be fancy or complicated: simple ingredients can create wonderful meals.

Have fun and stay connected.

- A positive attitude can change your whole outlook. Instead of looking at meal prep or cooking as a chore, make it fun. Turn on some music or get the family involved.
- Make physical activity a daily routine. Take a walk with a neighbor, or walk to the coffee shop. Take a hike with your friends instead of meeting for drinks. Try a dance class, or start a fitness challenge with friends. Find something you love doing and fit it into your life.
- Enjoy more meals with others. Make time for those long, leisurely dinners where no one is rushing, the conversation flows easily and the food is full of fresh ingredients.
- Share your new Mediterranean-inspired lifestyle with others. Share a recipe with a coworker or throw a Mediterranean-themed dinner party.

Now that you're prepped for success and ready to embark on your Mediterranean diet journey, I cannot wait for you to make, try and share the following recipes. From my home to yours—enjoy!

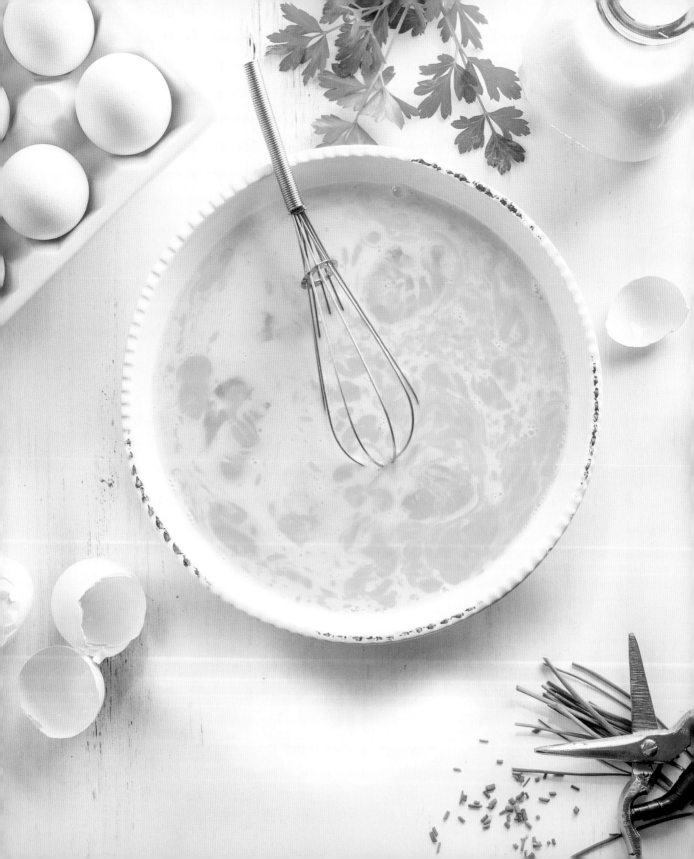

Nourishing MORNING MEALS

A few years ago, my husband and I stayed at a charming Airbnb outside of Florence, Italy. It was owned and renovated by a lovely couple who turned it into a picturesque home with beautiful views—complete with an outdoor kitchen and dining area.

On our second day there, the owner of the home made breakfast in the patio's wood-fired oven for all the guests. He called it "breakfast pie" and it was similar to a quiche. Golden brown, flaky crust surrounding fluffy eggs topped with tomatoes and herbs . . . it was delicious. The ingredients were simple, but they stood out because they were fresh and local: The eggs were fresh from the chickens. The tomatoes had been grown in the garden just steps down from the patio. The herbs were snipped from the assorted pots scattered around the yard.

When I returned back home after that trip, I made a conscious effort to try and re-create some of that magic in my everyday meals. I found that simple things— such as adding a few sliced tomatoes to scrambled eggs or adding a ripe, summer peach to a bowl of Greek yogurt—woke up my taste buds and left me feeling more satisfied than a bowl of sugary cereal or a highly-processed pastry.

In the Mediterranean diet, the focus of a typical breakfast is to create a balanced meal that you enjoy and that will fuel your body by including fresh fruit, whole grains, protein and fiber-rich foods. It doesn't have to be anything fancy or time consuming to prepare, especially because the mornings are a hectic time for many of us. The breakfast recipes in this chapter include easy weekday meals such as the Grab-and-Go Chocolate Chia Smoothie (page 32) or Cinnamon-Apple Slow Cooker Oats (page 39).

There are also a few recipes that take a little extra time and are perfect for slow-paced mornings or weekends, like the Hearty Breakfast Sandwich with Romesco Sauce (page 24). The ingredients are flexible, meaning you can substitute the fruit or vegetable in the recipe with another that's in season or something you enjoy more. But just as important as the ingredients is the notion of carving out a few minutes to actually savor your meal.

In addition to enjoying the recipes in this book, I encourage you to take a look at what you typically eat for breakfast. Ask yourself how you can add in a serving of fruit or vegetables, more whole grains or a bit of protein. Maybe that means tossing a handful of spinach in your scrambled eggs or adding fresh berries to your yogurt. Choose whole-grain bread for your toast or add peanut butter to your bagel in place of butter. Making small changes to the dishes you already enjoy is a simple way to start a Mediterranean-inspired diet.

SPICY SHAKSHUKA SKILLET

MAKES 4 SERVINGS

This is one of those dishes that looks fancy but is actually quite easy to make. It features eggs that are poached in a spicy tomato sauce flavored with warming spices such as cumin and paprika. The best part is breaking into the egg and having the perfectly runny yolk mix in with the tomato sauce. It will have you reaching for extra bread or a piece of Homemade Garlic and Herb Flatbread (page 45) to soak up all the delicious flavors.

2 tbsp (30 ml) extra virgin olive oil

1 bell pepper, diced

1 tsp ground cumin

1 tsp paprika

1 tsp red pepper flakes

½ tsp cayenne pepper

2 cloves garlic, minced

3 tbsp (56 g) tomato paste

1 (28-oz [794-g]) can plum tomatoes with liquid

5 large eggs

¼ cup (38 g) crumbled feta cheese

2 tbsp (8 g) chopped fresh Italian parsley

Preheat the oven to 400°F (200°C, or gas mark 6).

In a large, ovenproof skillet, heat the olive oil over medium heat. Once warm, add the bell pepper, cumin, paprika, red pepper flakes and cayenne pepper. Stir to combine and sauté for 5 minutes. Add the garlic and sauté, while stirring, for 1 minute.

Add the tomato paste and give a quick stir to combine before adding the plum tomatoes. Allow the mixture to come to a strong simmer before reducing the heat to low. Simmer the tomato sauce for 15 minutes, until it becomes thick and creamy. Make a divot in the sauce with the back of a wooden spoon and crack 1 egg directly into the divot. Repeat this process for all 5 of the eggs.

Carefully move the skillet to the oven and bake for 5 minutes, just until the eggs start to set, meaning they no longer wiggle when the pan moves and the whites of the egg are no longer transparent. If you prefer your eggs less runny, add 1 minute to the cook time. Remove the skillet from the oven and allow it to cool slightly before topping with the feta cheese and parsley.

TIP: Choose low-sodium or no-salt-added canned tomatoes whenever possible to reduce sodium intake. The combination of spices and feta cheese are flavorful enough that you won't even miss the salt.

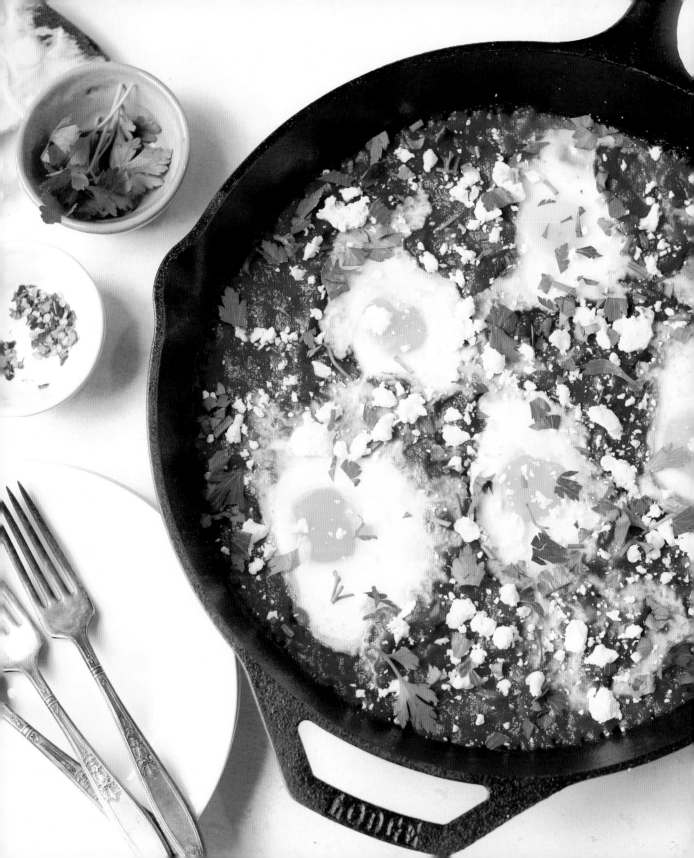

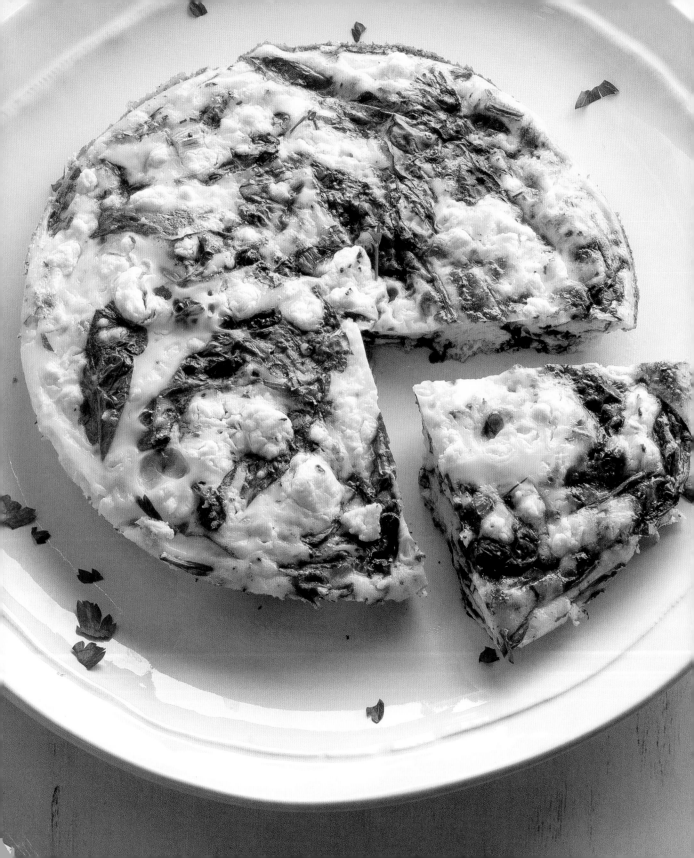

MAKE-AHEAD SPINACH *and* GOAT CHEESE FRITTATA

MAKES 6 TO 8 SERVINGS

Similar to a crustless quiche, a frittata is an egg-based dish that starts out on the stove and is finished in the oven. It is filling without being heavy and can be made in advance for a quick weekday breakfast. The beauty of this frittata recipe is you can easily change the vegetables based on what you have on hand or what's in season. Bell peppers, asparagus, arugula or fresh tomatoes are some of my favorite additions.

8 eggs

2 tbsp (30 ml) milk

¼ cup (25 g) grated Parmesan cheese

1 tbsp (4 g) chopped fresh Italian parsley

1 tbsp (3 g) chopped fresh chives

¼ tsp salt

¼ tsp pepper

2 tbsp (30 ml) extra virgin olive oil

1 medium shallot, thinly sliced

1 clove garlic, minced

8 oz (227 g) spinach

2 oz (60 g) goat cheese

Start by positioning a rack in the center of the oven. Preheat the oven to 375°F (190°C, or gas mark 5).

In a large bowl, whisk together the eggs, milk, Parmesan cheese, parsley, chives, salt and pepper. Set the bowl aside.

In a 10- to 12-inch (25- to 30-cm) nonstick, ovenproof skillet, heat the olive oil over medium heat. Once warm, add the shallot and sauté until it becomes translucent, about 3 to 4 minutes. Be sure to stir often. Add the garlic and sauté for 30 to 45 seconds.

Add the spinach to the pan. It will look like a lot of spinach, but once it starts wilting it becomes considerably smaller. Stir until all the spinach is wilted, about 45 to 60 seconds. Turn off the heat and carefully pour the contents of your skillet into the bowl with the eggs. Softly stir and then pour the egg-and-spinach mixture back into your skillet. Sprinkle the goat cheese over the top.

Place the skillet on the center rack of the oven. Cook the frittata for 12 to 14 minutes, just until the eggs in the center are set. Carefully remove the frittata from the oven and allow it to cool slightly. Cut into wedges to serve.

TIP: If you are typically a sausage/bacon person in the morning, adding chopped mushrooms is an easy way to make this dish even heartier without adding meat.

HEARTY BREAKFAST SANDWICH *with* ROMESCO SAUCE

MAKES 1 SERVING

Saturday morning bagels are a weekend tradition at my house that I always look forward to. This recipe is an easy, make-at-home version that is packed with crispy cucumber slices, fluffy eggs, creamy avocado and flavor-packed Romesco sauce. The end result is a hearty and filling breakfast that jump-starts your day with a bit of protein, fiber and healthy fats.

Choosing a whole-grain bagel will add some heart-healthy fiber and leave you feeling full longer. Feel free to add even more veggies, such as roasted bell peppers or fresh spinach, to change up the flavor profile. This bagel sandwich recipe also makes a great lunch dish. If you don't have Romesco sauce, creamy hummus also tastes great or even just mashed avocado with a bit of lemon juice.

1 bagel

1 tsp extra virgin olive oil

1 egg lightly beaten

1 tbsp (15 ml) Vibrant Romesco Sauce (page 181)

¼ cup (3 g) sprouts

3 slices cucumber

½ avocado, sliced

Slice your bagel and place it in the toaster. While your bagel is toasting, heat the olive oil in a small skillet over medium heat. Add the egg and scramble until cooked.

Spread the Romesco sauce evenly over your toasted bagel, then top with sprouts, scrambled egg, cucumber and avocado. Top with the remaining bagel half.

TIP: Romesco is a bell pepper and tomato sauce that adds a rich and slightly smoky flavor. It's simple to make yourself and store in the fridge. Check out my favorite romesco sauce recipe on page 181. You can also find romesco sauce in many grocery stores.

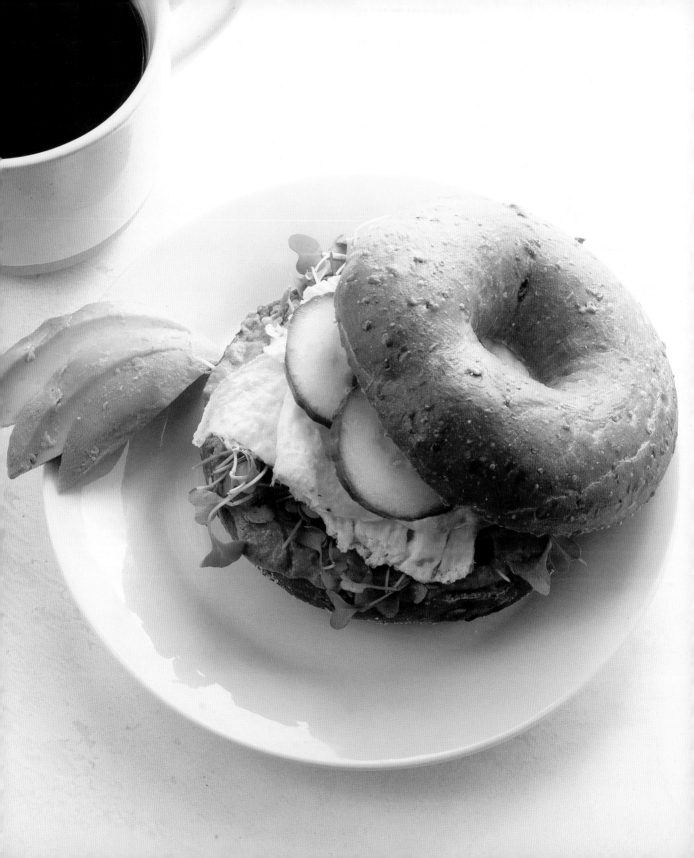

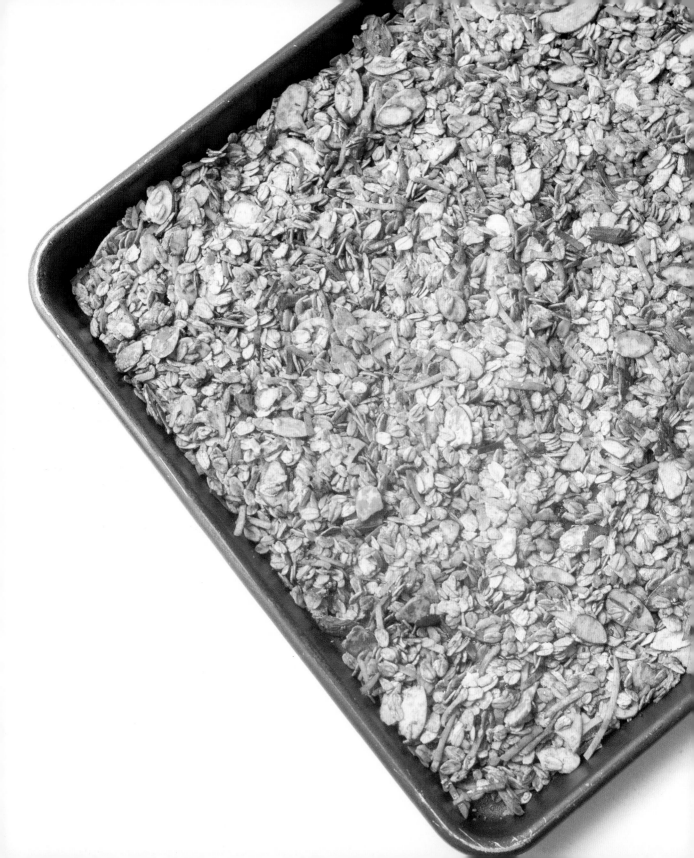

CRUNCHY CHOCOLATE-COCONUT GRANOLA

MAKES 4 CUPS (510 G)

Homemade granola can seem intimidating, but it's quite easy to make. This recipe is lightly sweetened with honey and real maple syrup, so it's not overly sweet and doesn't have all the added sugars that store-bought granola can sometimes contain. The chia seeds are a good source of heart-healthy omega-3 fatty acids, as well as a bit of protein, iron and magnesium.

In addition to just munching on this granola by itself, it tastes amazing on top of a bowl of creamy Greek yogurt, served with fresh fruit or even sprinkled on ice cream.

3 cups (270 g) rolled oats

1 cup (108 g) sliced almonds

1 cup (93 g) unsweetened coconut flakes

2 tbsp (25 g) chia seeds

2 tsp (2 g) ground cinnamon

1 tbsp (7 g) unsweetened cocoa powder

¼ cup (60 ml) honey

¼ tsp salt

¼ cup (60 ml) extra virgin olive oil

2 tbsp (30 ml) maple syrup

Start by preheating the oven to 250°F (120°C, or gas mark ½). Line a large baking sheet with parchment paper. You may need to use two pans to fit everything in a single layer.

In a large bowl, combine the rolled oats, almonds, coconut flakes, chia seeds, cinnamon and cocoa powder. Stir all the dry ingredients together until well combined.

Add the honey, salt, olive oil and maple syrup to the dry ingredients. The mixture will be a bit sticky, so use a rubber spatula to carefully mix all the ingredients together.

Spread the granola mixture in a thin layer on your parchment-lined baking sheet. Place the baking sheet in the oven and bake for 45 to 60 minutes. Stir the granola every 20 minutes to ensure it cooks evenly.

Once the granola is done, it will be golden brown and crisp. Allow it to cool completely before breaking the granola up into small chunks.

BREAKFAST GRAZING PLATE

Makes 1 serving

This recipe is a play on a Turkish breakfast, which is typically a light assortment of vegetables, bread, jams, cheese, olives and meats. The beauty of this grazing plate is that it's made up of simple foods you may already have on hand in the fridge or pantry. It's full of flavor, fills you up and creates a well-balanced meal that comes together quickly.

You can also completely customize this based on what you have on hand or the foods you like best. For example, swap out the cucumber and tomato for leftover roasted veggies from the night before, or add a little bit of yogurt topped with fresh fruit for a sweet component. This plate is perfect for anyone who is new to the Mediterranean diet or who prefers a light and simple breakfast.

2 hard-boiled eggs

1 small tomato, cut into quarters

¼ small cucumber, sliced

¼ cup (54 g) olives

2 tbsp (19 g) crumbled feta cheese

1 slice Herb-Baked Focaccia with Olives (page 50)

Arrange the eggs, tomato, cucumber, olives, feta and focaccia on a small platter or large plate.

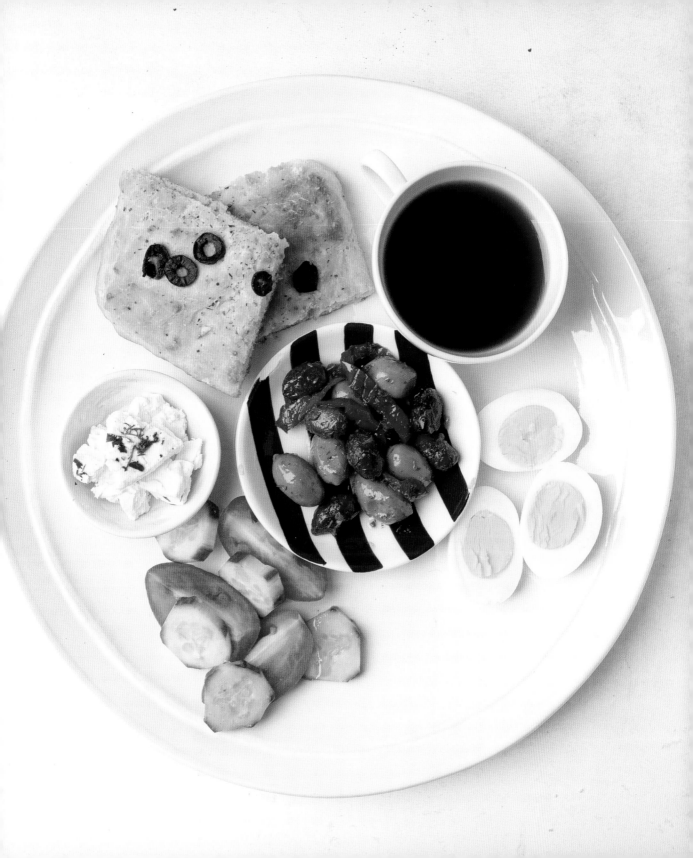

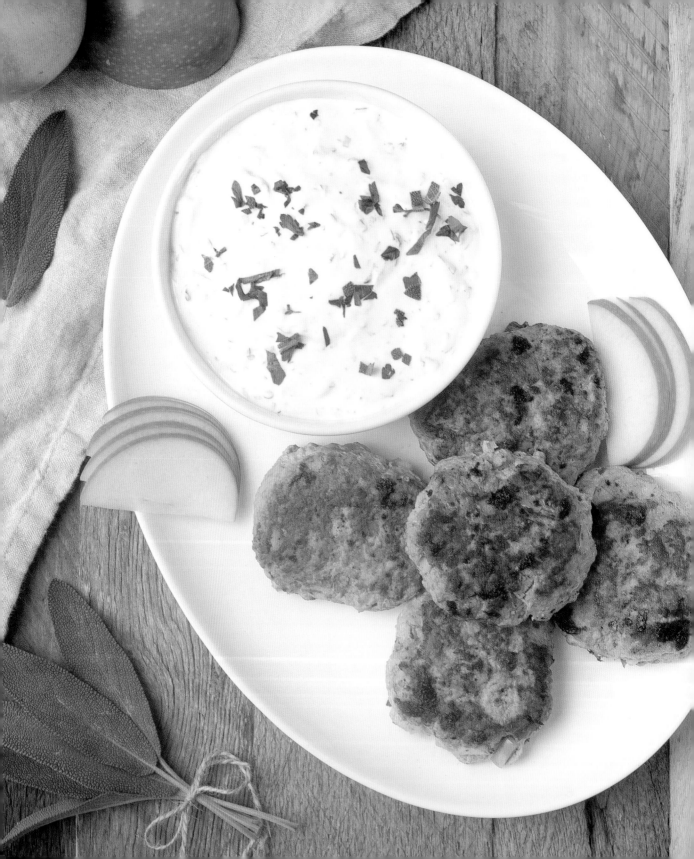

SAVORY TURKEY-APPLE SAUSAGE PATTIES *with* HERBED YOGURT

MAKES 4 LARGE PATTIES AND ½ CUP (120 ML) YOGURT

These turkey patties have such a warm, vibrant flavor. Made with lean ground turkey, fresh herbs and crisp apples, they are a healthy way to start the day. The star of the show is the herbed yogurt. It's creamy and tangy with just a hint of sage and lemon. If you are making these patties in advance, wait until serving to add the herbed yogurt.

HERBED YOGURT

½ cup (120 ml) plain Greek yogurt

2 tbsp (5 g) chopped fresh basil

1 tsp chopped fresh sage

½ tsp chopped fresh Italian parsley

1 clove garlic, minced

½ tsp fresh lemon juice

Salt and pepper, to taste

TURKEY-APPLE SAUSAGE

1 lb (454 g) ground turkey

½ cup (75 g) minced green apple

1 tsp chopped fresh sage

¼ tsp garlic powder

¼ tsp onion powder

¼ tsp salt

¼ tsp pepper

1 tbsp (15 ml) extra virgin olive oil

To make the herbed yogurt: Combine the Greek yogurt, basil, sage, parsley, garlic and lemon juice in a small bowl. Taste and add salt and pepper as needed. Cover the bowl and set it aside in the fridge.

To make the turkey-apple sausage: In a mixing bowl, combine the ground turkey with the apple, sage, garlic powder, onion powder, salt and pepper. Mix it all together with your hands or a spoon and form into four equal-sized patties.

To cook the turkey sausage patties, heat the olive oil in a large sauté pan over medium-high heat. Once warm, carefully place the four patties in the pan and cook until the turkey is cooked through, about 4 to 5 minutes on each side. Remove the turkey patties from the pan and top with the herbed yogurt.

TIP: Save any extra herbed yogurt in the fridge to use as a dip for raw veggies.

GRAB-*and*-GO CHOCOLATE CHIA SMOOTHIE

MAKES 2 (6-OUNCE [180-ML]) SMOOTHIES

Smoothies are a time-saver on busy mornings. They are also a great way to start your day off with a healthy dose of fruit, a bit of protein and some heart-healthy fats. This tastes like a rich, decadent treat, but it is actually full of wholesome ingredients. The frozen banana gives the smoothie a creamy texture while the chia seeds and almond butter provide the protein and the cocoa powder adds a hint of chocolate without the need for added sugars.

1 cup (240 ml) milk

1 tbsp (12 g) chia seeds

1 frozen banana

2 tbsp (60 g) almond butter

2 tbsp (14 g) unsweetened cocoa powder

1 tsp vanilla extract

Sliced banana, for garnish (optional)

In a high-powered blender, combine the milk, chia seeds, banana, almond butter, cocoa powder and vanilla. Puree until smooth and creamy.

Pour into two glasses and garnish with banana, if desired.

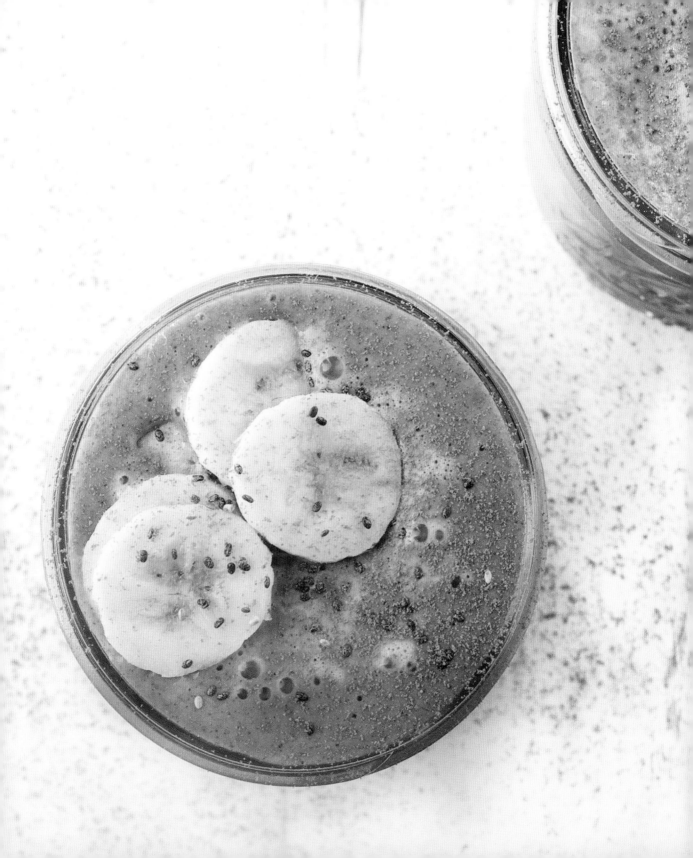

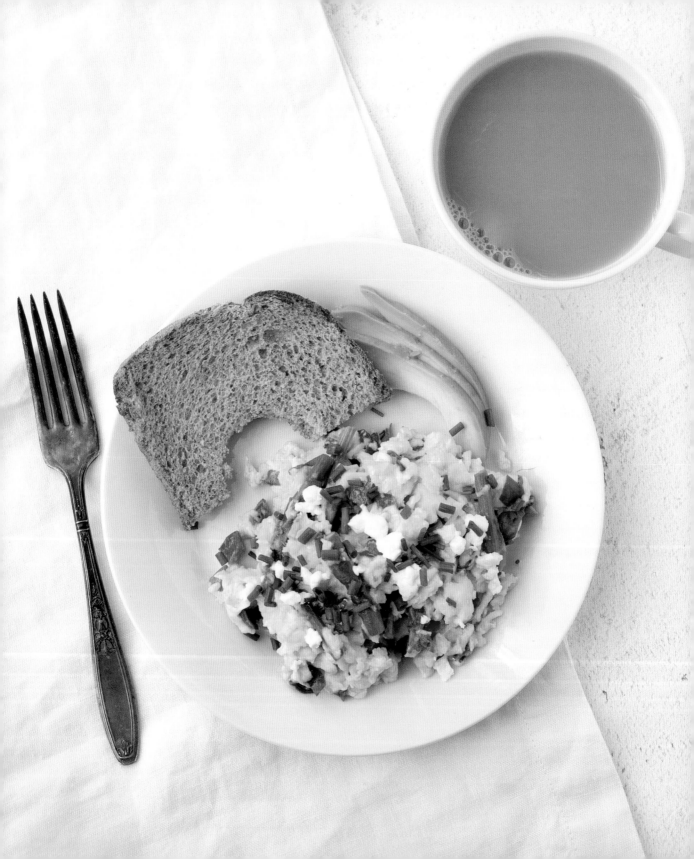

GREEN GARDEN SCRAMBLE

MAKES 2 SERVINGS

Scrambled eggs may seem like a plain recipe, but they are such a simple way to create a balanced, flavorful breakfast that doesn't take a lot of time to make. They are also a blank canvas for different flavor profiles and a great way to add some veggies to your morning meal.

This version takes some of my favorite green vegetables, fresh herbs and a bit of goat cheese to create a fresh meal that is perfect for sharing. It comes together quickly and can be served family style, making it the perfect meal to enjoy with company. You can easily substitute the vegetables for other favorites.

1 tbsp (15 ml) extra virgin olive oil

½ cup (65 g) chopped asparagus

½ cup (75 g) diced bell pepper

1 tsp garlic powder

6 eggs, lightly whisked in a bowl

1 cup (30 g) roughly chopped spinach

1 tbsp (3 g) chopped fresh chives

1 oz (25 g) goat cheese

Sliced avocado and sprouts, for serving (optional)

In a large skillet, heat the olive oil over medium heat. Once warm, add the asparagus, bell pepper and garlic powder. Lightly sauté until the vegetables are soft, about 4 to 5 minutes.

To the same skillet, add the eggs. Stir constantly with a wooden spoon or rubber spatula until the eggs are fully cooked, about 2 to 3 minutes. During the last minute, toss in the spinach and stir it into the eggs.

Top with the chives and goat cheese. Garnish with the avocado and sprouts, if desired.

ZESTY ZA'ATAR AVOCADO TOAST *with* POACHED EGG

MAKES 1 SERVING

This recipe calls for harissa, a chili pepper paste that is common throughout the Middle East. It's pretty spicy, so you only need to use a little bit. This dish also features one of my favorite Mediterranean spices—za'atar. It's an extremely aromatic spice blend that's earthy and flavorful, and I love adding it to so many recipes.

If you haven't poached an egg before, it isn't as difficult as it sounds. Though poaching an egg takes a little longer than scrambling or frying, I prefer a poached egg for this dish because it fits perfectly on the toast and makes the dish a bit more fun.

1 avocado, pitted and peeled

2 tbsp (30 ml) fresh lemon juice

1 tsp za'atar, divided

1 egg (The freshest egg possible is best here.)

1 tbsp (15 ml) white vinegar

1 slice whole-grain bread

1 tbsp (15 ml) harissa

Fresh basil, for garnish

Start by placing the avocado in a small bowl. Mash it with the back of a fork. Add the lemon juice and ½ teaspoon of the za'atar, and stir to combine. Set it aside.

Line a plate with a paper towel. Crack the egg into a small ramekin and set it aside. Fill a medium saucepot with 3 cups (720 ml) of water and bring to a boil over high heat. Once the water is boiling, reduce the heat to low and add the white vinegar. Use a spoon to stir the water, creating a small whirlpool in the pot. Carefully pour the egg directly from the ramekin into the center of the swirling water. Once the egg is in the pot, put your bread in the toaster while the egg cooks.

Allow the egg to cook for 3 minutes for a runny egg yolk. If you like a more well-done egg, add another minute of cooking time. Once the egg is finished, remove it from the water with a slotted spoon and transfer it to the lined plate.

While your egg cools slightly, spread the avocado mixture over your toasted slice of bread. Spread the harissa over the avocado and sprinkle with the remaining za'atar. Place the poached egg on top of the avocado toast, and garnish with a little bit of fresh basil.

TIP: Harissa is sold at many chain grocery stores and online. If you can't find it, substitute hot sauce or regular chili paste.

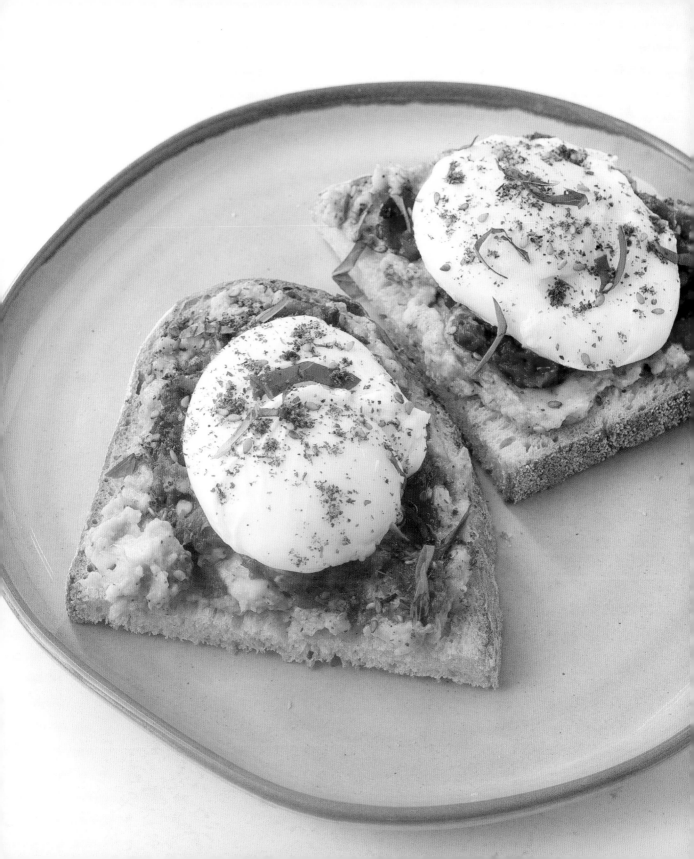

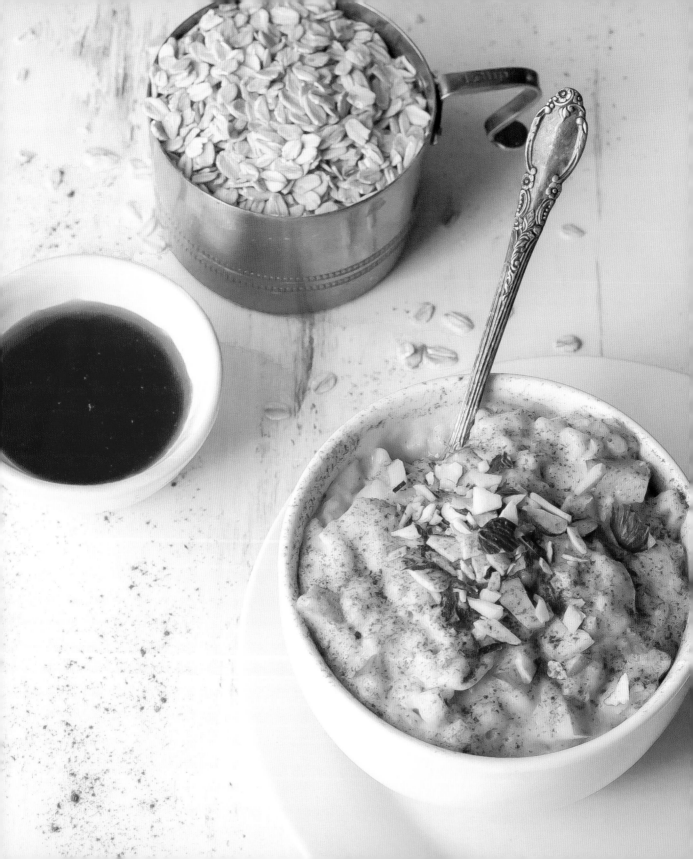

CINNAMON-APPLE SLOW COOKER OATS

MAKES 3 SERVINGS

This slow cooker recipe is a great example of how to take a common breakfast dish and apply some of the Mediterranean diet guidelines by adding fresh fruit, using spices for flavor and keeping the ingredients simple. The end result is a thick and creamy breakfast that warms you from the inside out.

Rolled oats are whole grains that are a good source of vitamins and minerals. They absorb the cooking liquid and become soft, tender and fluffy when finished. Lightly sweetened with fresh apples and a hint of maple syrup, this dish is not overly sweet. If you like a little extra sweetness, feel free to add a bit more maple syrup or top it with a drizzle of honey or additional fresh fruit.

1 cup (90 g) rolled oats

1½ cups (360 ml) milk

1 apple, peeled, cored and diced

1 tbsp (15 ml) maple syrup

1 tsp ground cinnamon

Add the oats, milk, 1½ cups (360 ml) of water, apple, maple syrup and cinnamon to your slow cooker. Stir to combine. Cook on low for 3 hours or high for 60 to 75 minutes.

Allow it to cool slightly before serving, or store in the fridge and simply reheat before enjoying.

TIP: Adding nuts and dried fruit to this oatmeal is also a great way to add even more of the Mediterranean diet principles to your breakfast. One of my favorites is adding chopped walnuts and unsweetened dried cranberries right before serving.

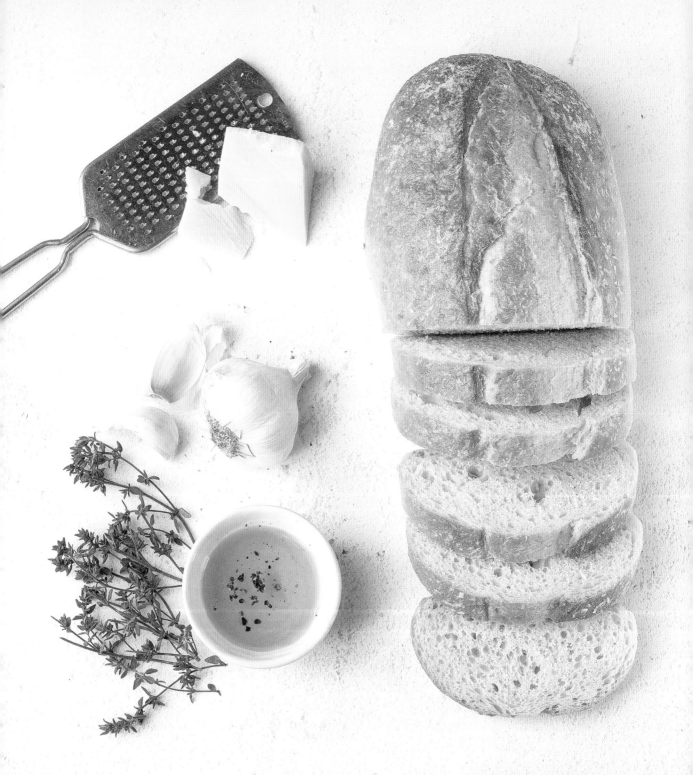

Appetizing SMALL PLATES

One of the hardest parts about making changes to your diet can be when food-related functions, such as parties or celebrations, are thrown into the mix. The goal of the Mediterranean diet is to create a long-term lifestyle, which means that all those dinner parties, baby showers and backyard barbecues are going to need to fit into your new way of eating.

The great news is that the Mediterranean diet isn't a list of dos and don'ts when it comes to food: You can feel completely comfortable enjoying dinner at a friend's house or attending a cocktail party.

The recipes in this chapter are delicious and shareable dishes that are inspired by popular party appetizers, but with a Mediterranean twist. Many of the recipes in this chapter feature fresh herbs, dried fruit or nuts and seeds to add big flavors and texture to the dishes. When cheese is used, it's often a variety with a strong flavor, such as feta or goat cheese, and only a small amount is needed.

These recipes feature simple ingredients that are transformed into crowd-pleasing favorites. The Warm Feta with Fresh Herbs (page 42) always gets devoured every single time I bring it to any function. If you've ever wanted to try your hand at making fresh bread, the Homemade Garlic and Herb Flatbread (page 45) is the perfect place to start. It's an easy recipe made with real ingredients, and it makes the most tender flatbread without all the kneading and rising time that traditional bread recipes require.

The goal of this chapter is to show you that you can still enjoy your favorite appetizers at parties and functions simply by incorporating a few more vegetables, fresh fruits, nuts, seeds or whole grains. Remember that the Mediterranean diet is designed to be a lifestyle that includes social interaction and the celebration of good food. So the next time you're invited to a get-together, you can feel confident whipping up one of these delicious dishes and sharing your healthy lifestyle with others.

WARM FETA *with* FRESH HERBS

MAKES 8 OUNCES (227 G)

This recipe is my play on the traditional "cheese plate" party appetizer. A light drizzle of olive oil and a sprinkle of red pepper flakes is all the prep this tangy feta needs before it's baked in the oven and becomes warm and creamy. The dish is finished off with plenty of fresh herbs for a bright and fresh small plate that tastes amazing with pita chips or sliced vegetables.

I typically serve this with cucumbers, but it also goes well with carrot sticks, sliced radishes or bell peppers. It is my go-to dish to bring to parties because it is easy to make and always a crowd favorite. It also makes a great accompaniment to a leisurely weekend lunch.

8 oz (227 g) feta block

1 tsp extra virgin olive oil

½ tsp red pepper flakes

½ tsp pepper

½ tbsp (2 g) chopped fresh dill

½ tbsp (2 g) chopped fresh Italian parsley

½ medium cucumber, sliced

1 cup (227 g) pita chips

Start by positioning a rack in the center of the oven. Preheat the oven to 400°F (200°C, or gas mark 6).

Pat your feta block lightly with a paper towel to remove any excess moisture. Brush each side of the feta with the olive oil and place it in an ovenproof baking dish. Sprinkle the top of the feta with red pepper flakes and pepper. Bake for 10 minutes.

Remove the feta from the oven and allow it to cool slightly before topping with the dill and parsley.

Serve with the cucumber and pita chips.

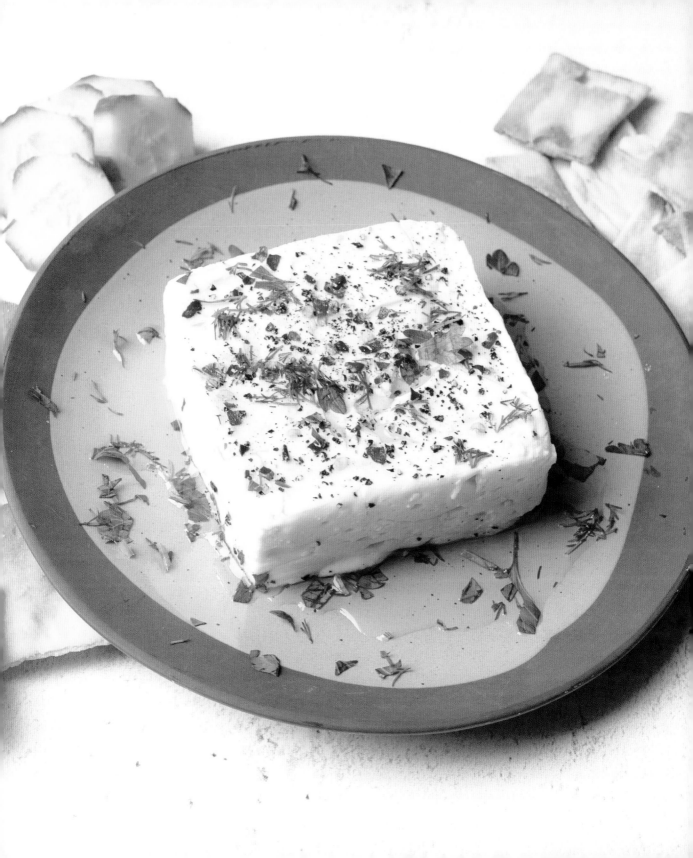

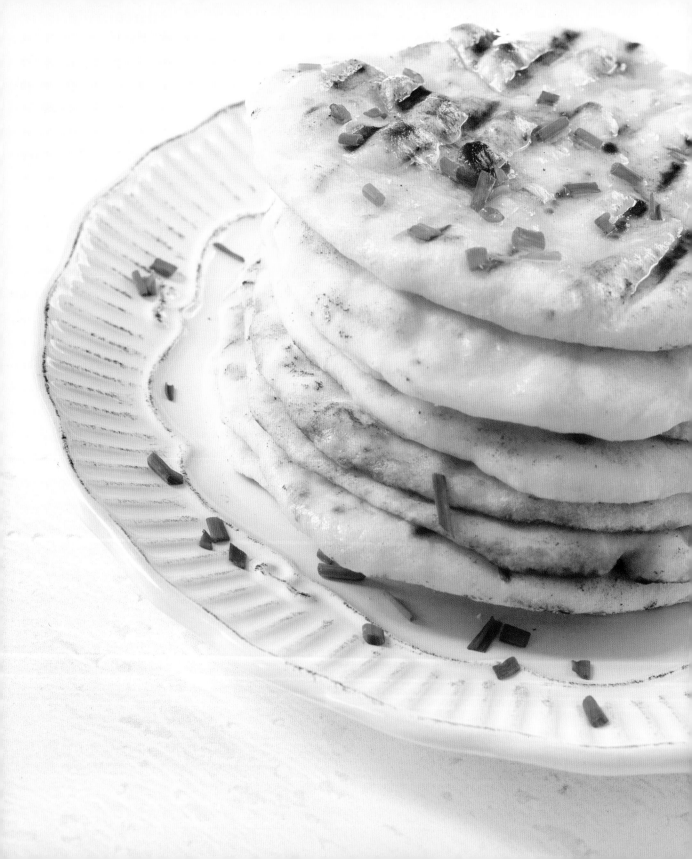

HOMEMADE GARLIC *and* HERB FLATBREAD

MAKES 8 SERVINGS

When I was in Greece, I couldn't get enough of the fresh, homemade flatbread they served at many restaurants. It was perfectly crisp on the outside and wonderfully tender and fluffy on the inside. After returning back home, I couldn't find anything similar, so I tried my hand at making it myself.

Turns out it's not difficult at all and the end result is the BEST flatbread ever. It's light, fluffy and made from real ingredients. The process does take a little time, but the end result is well worth the effort. My kids love helping me make this recipe, which also makes it a fun family activity that hopefully they'll pass on to their kids.

1 (¼-oz [7-g]) package active dry yeast

2 cloves garlic, minced

2 tbsp (6 g) minced fresh chives

½ tsp salt

½ tsp sugar

2 cups (250 g) all-purpose flour (plus additional for flouring the work surface)

1 tbsp (15 ml) extra virgin olive oil

In a large mixing bowl, combine the yeast, garlic, chives, salt, sugar and flour. Whisk the dry ingredients together until well combined.

Make a well in the center of the flour mixture and add ½ cup (120 ml) of lukewarm water; be sure the water is not too hot or you will kill the yeast. Add the olive oil. Using a wooden spoon, stir gently to mix all the ingredients together. Slowly add more water as needed—up to ¼ cup (60 ml)—until a sticky dough forms.

Lightly flour a clean work surface and gently transfer your dough onto the surface. Using the palms of your hands, gently knead the dough until it becomes smooth and elastic, about 2 minutes. Softly form it into a ball.

Wipe out your original mixing bowl and place your dough in the center, seam side down. Cover with a damp tea towel and place in a warm place to rise for 1 hour. After an hour, the dough will double in size. Remove the dough from the bowl and cut into eight equal pieces; I use a pair of scissors.

Roll each piece into a ball and then gently flatten into a flat circle. Allow the dough to rest while you heat a cast-iron skillet over medium-high heat. Once warm, cook each flatbread one at a time for about 2 minutes each side, just until the outside is golden brown. Remove the flatbread and allow it to cool slightly before use.

DELICIOUSLY EASY GOAT CHEESE APRICOTS

MAKES 2 DOZEN

Having people over for meals is such a fun way to connect with loved ones. What isn't fun is the stress that can come with getting everything pulled together before people arrive.

This easy appetizer recipe is my perfect solution to that problem. This dish comes together so quickly and can be made in advance. The best part is . . . people love them! Made with dried apricots and pistachios, they offer a bit of fiber and heart-healthy fats, which makes them filling without being heavy. I use goat cheese because it has such a strong, tangy flavor, so only a tiny bit is needed in each apricot bite.

2 oz (60 g) herbed goat cheese, at room temperature

24 dried apricots

¼ cup (31 g) chopped pistachios

Place a small spoonful of herbed goat cheese on each of the dried apricots. Sprinkle each apricot with pistachios, and place them on a serving platter.

If you are making these in advance, store them in the fridge and allow the dish to come to room temperature before serving.

TIP: If fresh apricots are in season, they can easily be substituted for the dried version in this recipe. Just cut them in half, remove the pit and top with a bit of goat cheese and the chopped pistachios. You may need to slightly increase the amount of goat cheese and pistachios used because whole apricots are a bit bigger than dried.

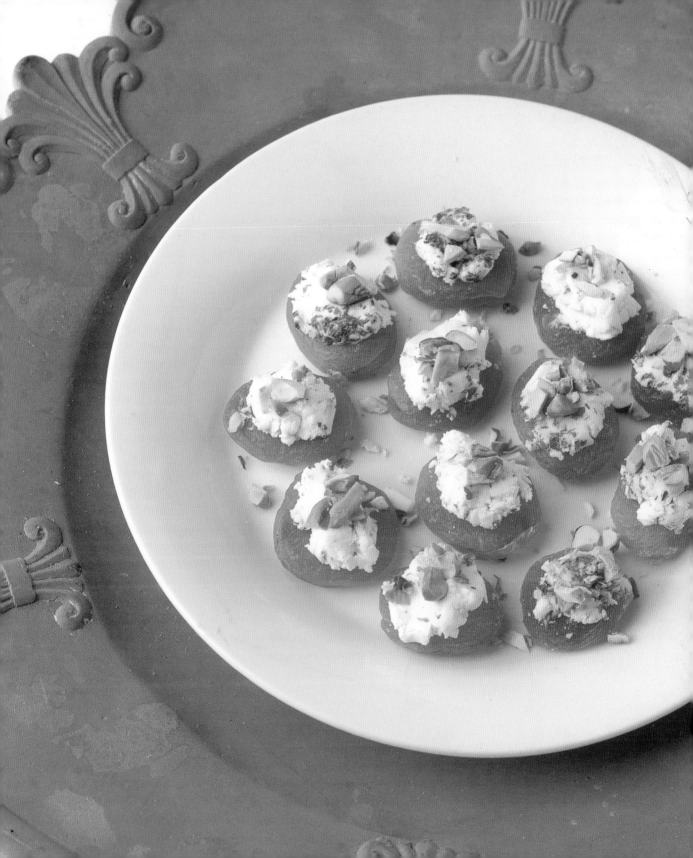

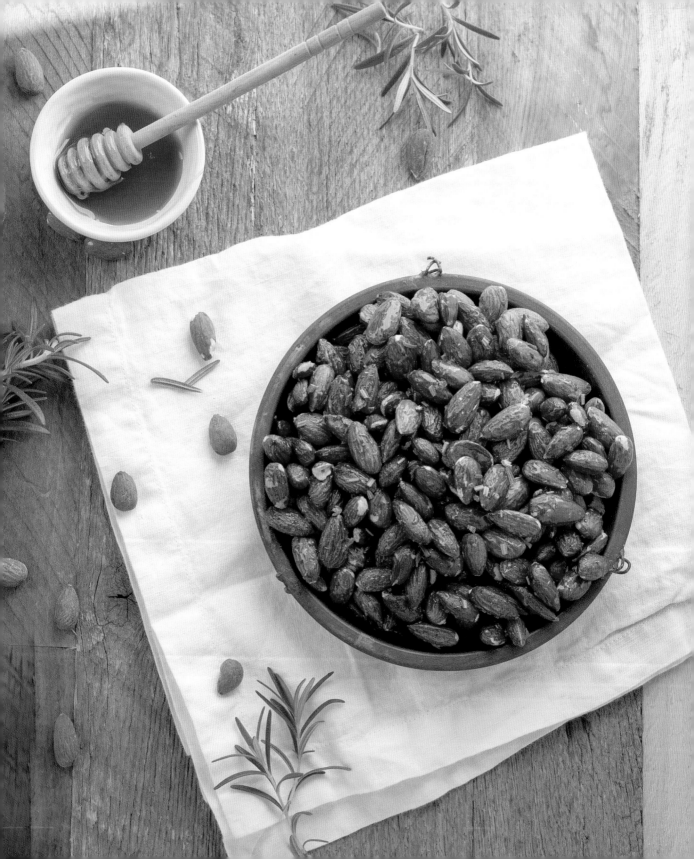

ROSEMARY *and* HONEY ROASTED ALMONDS

MAKES 2 CUPS (294 G)

Whenever we had people over, my mom usually put out a bowl of honey-roasted peanuts for our guests. It was one of my favorite parts of having company over. To this day, I still love snacking on nuts, and this recipe turns that traditional bowl of honey-roasted nuts into a slightly sweet and savory, heart-healthy snack. I replaced the peanuts with almonds for a bit of protein and flavored them with plenty of fresh rosemary, garlic and bit of honey for sweetness.

2 cups (286 g) raw almonds

1 tbsp (15 ml) extra virgin olive oil

1 tbsp (2 g) minced fresh rosemary

1 clove garlic, minced

¼ tsp salt

1 tbsp (15 ml) honey

Start by preheating the oven to 300°F (150°C, or gas mark 2). Line a baking sheet with parchment paper.

Spread the almonds in a single layer on the baking sheet. Roast the almonds in the oven for 15 minutes, shaking them halfway through to ensure they roast evenly. Remove the almonds from the oven and turn the temperature down to 200°F (93°C).

In a large skillet over medium heat, add the olive oil and rosemary and sauté for 2 minutes, stirring constantly. Add the garlic and sauté for 30 seconds, just until the garlic becomes fragrant. To the same pan, add the salt and roasted almonds. Stir to combine. Add the honey to the almond mixture and stir.

Spread the honey-almond mixture back onto your parchment-lined baking sheet in an even, single layer. Place the baking sheet back in the oven and roast for 15 to 20 minutes.

Remove the baking sheet from the oven and allow the almonds to cool slightly before serving.

HERB-BAKED FOCACCIA *with* OLIVES

There is a French bakery near me that sells the most heavenly sourdough baguettes that have people lining up around the block every Saturday. They often sell out quickly and people ask the owner why she doesn't just make more. Her response is always "because enough is enough." If she made more, then people would purchase too many or it wouldn't be special anymore.

This same sentiment can be applied to the Mediterranean diet. Enjoying high-quality, homemade bread, for example, is a special treat to be enjoyed immensely. But it's not necessarily an everyday occasion. This baked focaccia recipe is a foolproof homemade bread recipe for those of us who aren't "bakers." Using a rapid rise yeast is my little shortcut for creating homemade bread without all the "waiting for it to rise" time. It isn't the same as active dry yeast, so be sure to purchase the right kind. The end result is freshly baked bread made with your own two hands and real ingredients.

3 cups (375 g) all-purpose flour

1 (¼-oz [7-g]) envelope rapid rise yeast

1 tbsp (15 g) sugar

1 tsp salt

4 tbsp (60 ml) extra virgin olive oil, divided

¼ cup (54 g) sliced Kalamata olives

1 tbsp (2 g) chopped fresh rosemary

Start by lightly greasing a 13 x 9–inch (33 x 23–cm) baking pan.

In a large bowl, mix together the flour, yeast, sugar and salt. Make a well in the center of the dry ingredients. Pour in 2 tablespoons (30 ml) of olive oil and 1⅔ cups (400 ml) of very warm water; be sure the water is not too hot or you will kill the yeast. Stir well, just until everything is combined and a sticky dough forms.

Spread the dough out into the greased baking pan and lightly press until it is evenly spread over the entire pan. Cover the dough with a damp dish towel and let it rise for 30 minutes.

Use the handle of a wooden spoon to push multiple holes into the dough. Drizzle the top of the dough with the remaining olive oil, and top it with the olives and rosemary. Cover the dough again and allow it to rise for 15 minutes.

While you are waiting for the dough to rise, position a rack in the center of the oven and preheat the oven to 375°F (190°C, or gas mark 5).

Once the dough has risen again, bake it for 30 minutes. Allow the focaccia to cool before serving. Leftovers can be covered well and saved at room temperature for about 3 to 5 days.

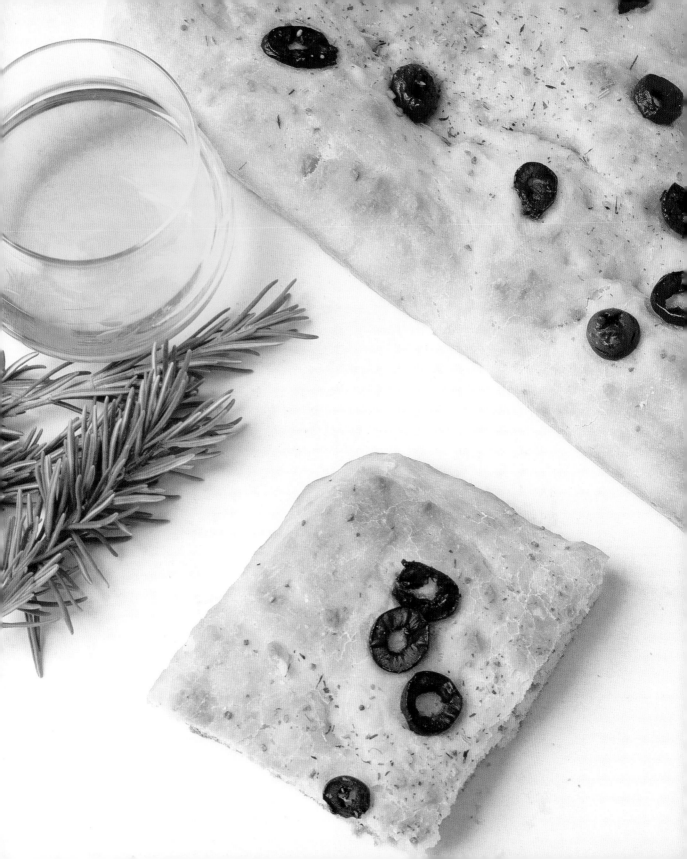

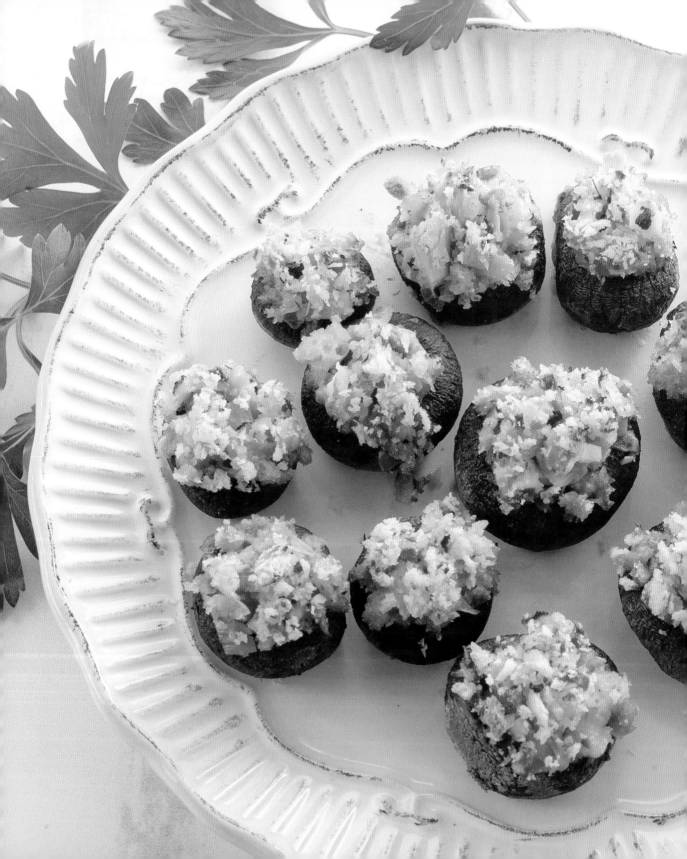

MOUTHWATERING STUFFED MUSHROOMS

I absolutely love stuffed mushrooms because there are so many different flavors you can pack into that tiny little mushroom cap. This recipe puts a Mediterranean spin on an old classic by adding the flavors of sautéed bell peppers, artichoke hearts and Greek seasoning. This recipe is completely vegetarian, but you'll never miss the meat because you add the chopped mushroom stems back into the stuffing mixture, making it hearty and earthy and oh so delicious.

16 oz (454 g) whole cremini or button mushrooms

1 tbsp (15 ml) extra virgin olive oil

1 medium bell pepper, seeds removed and diced

½ medium onion, diced

2 cloves garlic, minced

¼ cup (34 g) canned artichoke hearts, drained and finely chopped

1 tsp Greek Seasoning Spice Blend (page 177)

½ cup (25 g) panko-style breadcrumbs

¼ cup (38 g) crumbled feta cheese

¼ cup (25 g) grated Parmesan cheese

Preheat the oven to 375°F (190°C, or gas mark 5). Line a large baking sheet with parchment paper.

Start by removing the stems from the mushrooms. Finely chop the removed stems and set them aside. In a large sauté pan, heat the olive oil over medium heat. Once the oil and pan are warm, add the mushroom stems, bell pepper, onion, garlic, artichoke hearts and Greek seasoning. Stir to combine and sauté for 5 to 6 minutes.

Remove the pan from the heat and place the sautéed mixture in a large mixing bowl to cool slightly. While the stuffing is cooling, line up the mushroom caps on the parchment-lined baking sheet.

Once the stuffing mixture is cooled, add the breadcrumbs, feta cheese and Parmesan cheese. Mix until everything is well combined.

Using a small spoon, fill each mushroom cap with the stuffing mixture until overflowing. Place the baking sheet in the oven and bake for about 20 minutes, until the mushrooms are cooked through and the stuffing mixture is golden brown.

QUICK *and* SIMPLE TORTELLINI BITES

MAKES 24 BITES

This stunning dish is like having the perfect bite of pasta in appetizer form. Each skewer contains a perfect balance of tortellini, bright cherry tomato, fresh basil and briny olives. A little drizzle of balsamic glaze brings the whole dish together but keeps it light and refreshing at the same time. The whole dish can be made in advance, making it perfect for parties.

2 cups (216 g) cheese tortellini

1 cup (150 g) cherry tomatoes

1 cup (180 g) green olives

2 tbsp (5 g) chopped fresh basil

¼ cup (60 ml) balsamic glaze, divided

Bring a large pot of water to a boil. Add the tortellini and cook until just done, about 6 to 7 minutes. Drain and set the tortellini aside to cool slightly.

Place two tortellini, a cherry tomato and a green olive on each long toothpick or skewer. Arrange on a platter and garnish with fresh basil. Drizzle the platter with about 2 tablespoons (30 ml) of balsamic glaze and place the rest in a small dipping bowl to serve alongside the appetizer. Guests can then add extra balsamic glaze, if desired.

If you are making this dish in advance, save the balsamic drizzle until just before serving.

TIP: The tortellini can be cooked in advance and stored in the fridge until ready to assemble. You can also customize the ingredients based on what's in season or what you have on hand. If it isn't tomato season, consider adding a piece of roasted bell pepper or canned artichoke heart instead.

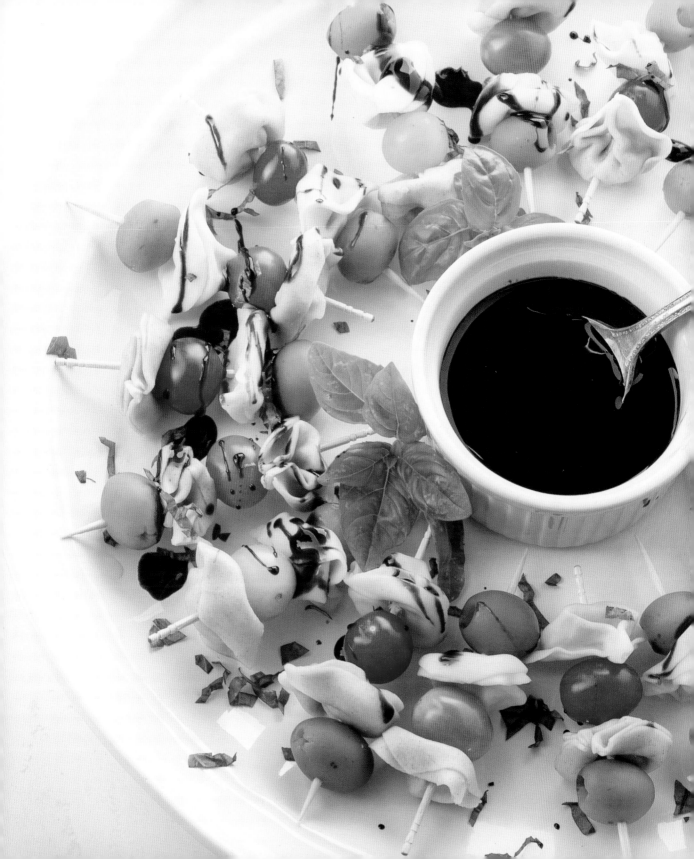

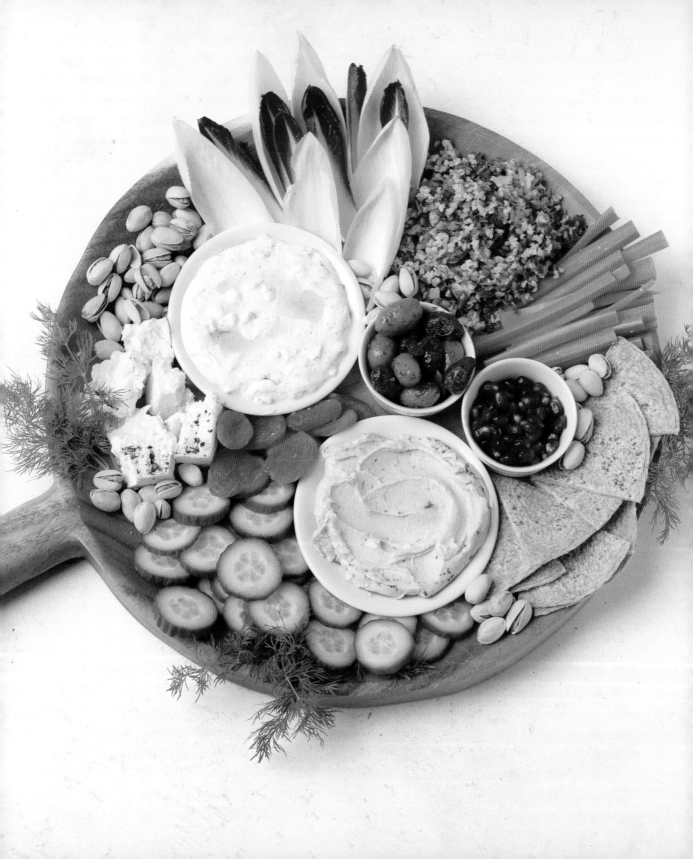

SHAREABLE MEZE PARTY PLATTER

MAKES 6 TO 8 SERVINGS

The word "meze" translates into "taste" or "snack" in Persian, and it is a huge part of the dining experience in many Mediterranean countries. Simply put, it's a collection of finger foods that can be hearty enough to become a meal.

This meze platter is a Mediterranean twist on the somewhat boring crudité platters of my generation. While still offering the traditional raw vegetables such as cucumbers and carrot sticks, the platter is updated a bit. Crispy endive offers the perfect vehicle for dipping into creamy hummus or tangy tzatziki. Dried apricots, tart pomegranate arils and crunchy pistachios offer plenty of different textures and easily snackable items. I serve mine with wedges of Homemade Garlic and Herb Flatbread (page 45), but you could also substitute with store-bought flatbread or pita bread to make it easier to put together.

1 medium cucumber, sliced into rounds

2 small carrots, peeled and cut into sticks

¼ cup (54 g) olives

1 cup (225 g) The Best Hummus with Lemon and Roasted Garlic (page 170)

1 cup (50 g) endive leaves

2 pieces Homemade Garlic and Herb Flatbread (page 45)

1 cup (240 ml) Traditional Tzatziki Sauce with Fresh Dill (page 166)

1 cup (227 g) Fresh Lemon and Herb Tabbouleh Salad (page 123)

2 tbsp (14 g) pomegranate arils

¼ cup (31 g) pistachios

¼ cup (35 g) dried apricots

Simply arrange the cucumber, carrots, olives, hummus, endive, flatbread, tzatziki, tabbouleh, pomegranate arils, pistachios and dried apricots on a large serving platter or cutting board.

TIP: Hummus, tzatziki and tabbouleh are often easy to find at most large chain or specialty grocery stores now. If you don't have time to make them yourself, try purchasing one that has the most "real-food" ingredients on the label.

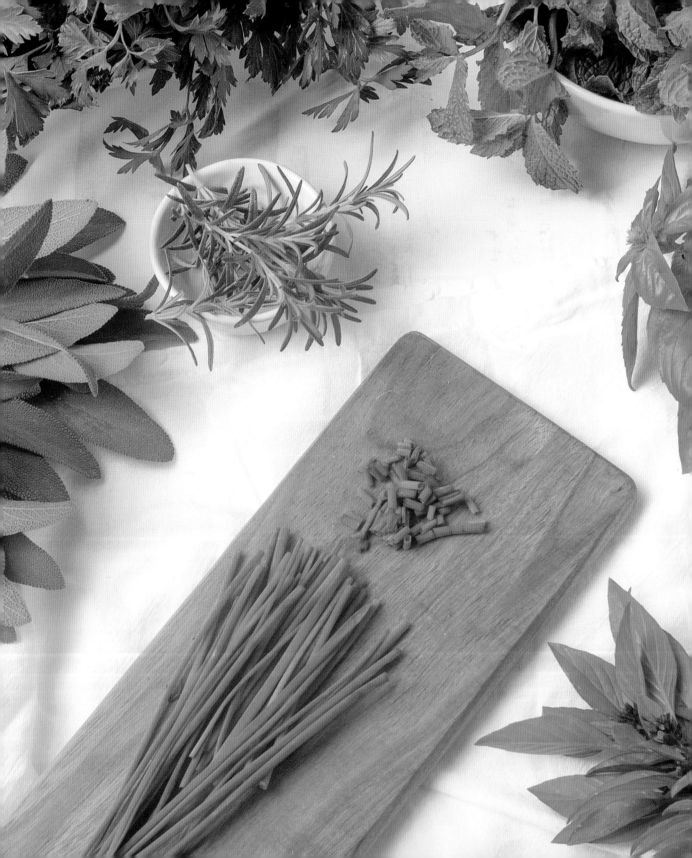

Filling and FLAVORFUL LUNCHES

I think that lunch may be one of the trickiest meals for many people, especially when they are trying to eat healthier. People either fall into the pitfall of trying to eat "light" by just having a salad (i.e., bowl of lettuce and veggies with dressing). Or they don't prepare anything and rely on grabbing a quick bite from the deli on the corner during their lunch break.

While adding veggies to your meals via a salad is an effort to be applauded, it can often leave you feeling unfulfilled, hungry and bored. Buying something on your lunch break can often mean limited choices and meals prepared with artificial ingredients or hidden sugars and saturated fats.

The filling and flavorful lunch recipes in this book offer bright, vibrant dishes that will have you looking forward to lunch all morning long. They are also balanced with fiber-filled vegetables, whole grains and legumes that are designed to offer great flavor and leave you feeling full and satisfied until your next meal. Sources of lean protein include everything from canned tuna and grilled shrimp to black beans and creamy hummus.

You'll see many of the dishes are flavored with lots of fresh herbs and spices, such as the Crispy Baked Falafel (page 64). Others are enhanced with lots of flavor and texture from nuts, seeds and dried fruit, such as the Sweet and Savory Apricot Couscous Salad (page 76). Most of the recipes can be prepared in advance: With just a little time set aside for meal prep, you can have your lunches ready to go during the busy week.

With all the stressors and constantly trying to do everything as quickly as possible in today's culture, I also challenge you to find the time to sit down for your lunch, even if it's just for fifteen minutes. Savor the dish you took the time to create, or put away your phone and engage in a conversation with a coworker in the break room. Remember that the foods we eat are only one part of trying to live a more Mediterranean-inspired lifestyle. Celebrating food and fostering social interactions is another crucial part to a more well-balanced lifestyle filled with the joy of sharing meals with others.

GARDEN FRESH GRILLED VEGETABLE SANDWICH

MAKES 2 SANDWICHES

Vegetable sandwiches often consist of a few soggy vegetables and don't have much flavor. This recipe creates a filling, satisfying sandwich that will prove to you that meatless meals don't have to be boring. The key is to season the veggies lightly before grilling to add flavor to each component of the sandwich. Using a homemade pesto as a sandwich spread adds so much flavor and complements the grilled vegetables perfectly. I prefer using zucchini and yellow squash because they hold up best when grilled, but you could easily substitute them for eggplant or even raw veggies.

Feel free to top the sandwich with even more flavor enhancers, such as fresh sliced tomatoes, creamy and filling avocado, fresh sprouts or pickles.

1 medium zucchini, cut lengthwise into ½-inch (1-cm) slices

1 medium yellow squash, cut lengthwise into ½-inch (1-cm) slices

1 bell pepper, seeded and cut into strips

1 tsp extra virgin olive oil

1 tsp dried basil

1 tsp dried oregano

4 slices whole wheat bread

2 tbsp (28 g) Peppery Arugula-Walnut Pesto (page 173)

1 cup (34 g) arugula

Warm a grill pan or large skillet over medium-high heat. While the pan is heating up, place the zucchini, squash and bell pepper in a large bowl. Drizzle the vegetables with the olive oil. Add the basil and oregano, and mix until well coated. Place the vegetables on the grill pan. Grill for about 3 to 4 minutes on each side.

While your vegetables are grilling, lightly toast the bread.

To assemble the sandwiches, spread the pesto on 2 of the slices of toasted bread. Evenly divide the arugula over the other slices of toasted bread. Top the arugula with the grilled vegetables and top it with the pesto-spread bread slice.

TIP: Pesto makes a flavorful dip for veggies, making it a simple way to help you eat and enjoy more vegetables.

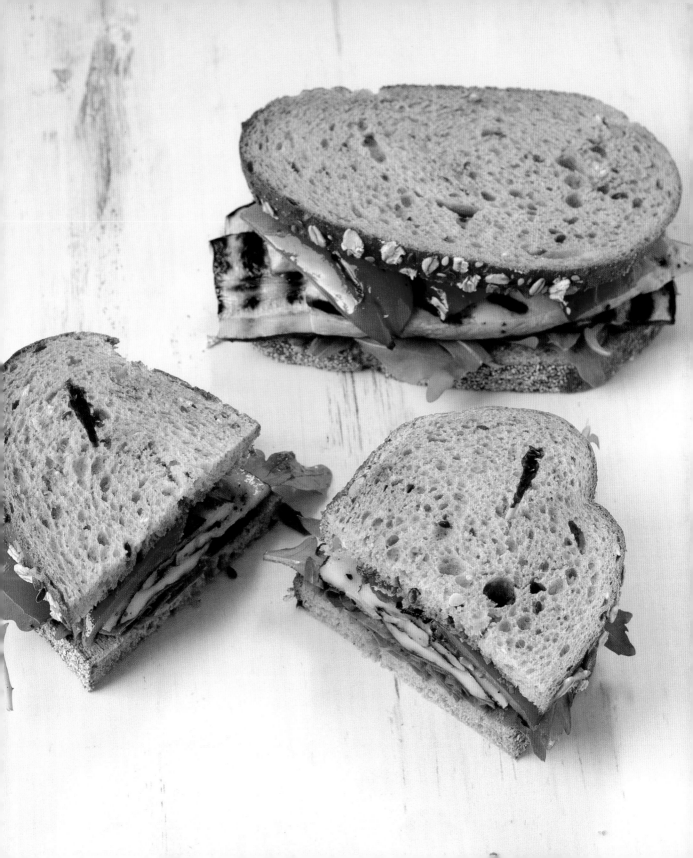

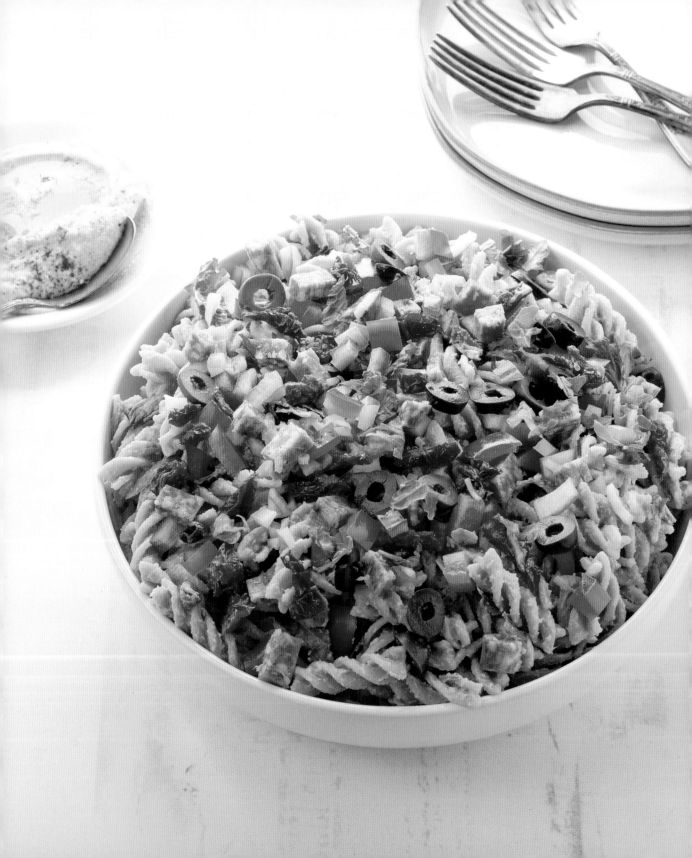

ZESTY PASTA SALAD *with* CREAMY HUMMUS DRESSING

MAKES 6 SERVINGS

The Greek restaurant near my house serves the best pasta salad. It's creamy and tangy, but it isn't substantial enough to serve as a stand-alone meal. This pasta salad recipe is inspired by the one served at the restaurant, but it's hearty enough to be a filling lunch. This salad is filled with crispy vegetables, sweet sun-dried tomatoes and tangy olives all tossed together with a creamy hummus dressing. The recipe calls for salami, but you could easily substitute that for grilled chicken, shrimp or even tofu if you're looking for a vegetarian option.

1 lb (454 g) whole wheat pasta

½ cup (113 g) The Best Hummus with Lemon and Roasted Garlic (page 170)

1 bell pepper, diced

¼ cup (40 g) diced red onion

2 oz (60 g) salami, cubed

1 cup (67 g) roughly chopped kale

¼ cup (21 g) sun-dried tomatoes

¼ cup (54 g) sliced Kalamata olives

Bring a large pot of water to a boil over medium heat. Add the pasta and cook until al dente, about 10 minutes. Drain the pasta and pour it into a large bowl.

Add the hummus and mix well to incorporate. When added to the warm pasta, it will naturally turn into a thick sauce that coats the pasta. Add the bell pepper, onion, salami, kale, sun-dried tomatoes and olives to the bowl. Mix until all the ingredients are combined.

CRISPY BAKED FALAFEL

MAKES 3 SERVINGS

Falafel is a flavorful blend of chickpeas and spices that are typically fried in oil until crispy. This version is baked, making it a bit easier to prepare, without sacrificing any of the amazing flavor and texture. Instead of the traditional pita that falafel is often served with, I've paired this recipe with creamy hummus, refreshing cucumber and tangy pomegranates. It's one of my favorite lunches, and it can easily be made in advance and taken to work or school.

1½ cups (360 g) canned chickpeas, drained and rinsed

½ cup (30 g) chopped fresh Italian parsley

½ cup (8 g) chopped fresh cilantro

½ cup (80 g) diced onion

3 cloves garlic, roughly chopped

1 tsp ground cumin

½ tsp salt

½ tsp pepper

2 tsp (10 ml) fresh lemon juice

2 tbsp (30 ml) extra virgin olive oil

2 cups (450 g) The Best Hummus with Lemon and Roasted Garlic (page 170)

½ cup (67 g) diced cucumber

¼ cup (27 g) pomegranate arils

Start by preheating the oven to 375°F (190°C, or gas mark 5). Line a baking sheet with parchment paper.

One of the keys to this recipe is making sure that the chickpeas are patted as dry as possible with a paper towel. This will help when you form them into patties.

In a food processor, add the parsley, cilantro, onion and garlic. Pulse until everything is finely chopped. Add the chickpeas, cumin, salt, pepper and lemon juice to the food processor. Pulse everything together until pureed. With the food processor still running, slowly add the olive oil, 1 tablespoon (15 ml) at a time. Only add enough olive oil to make the falafel mixture creamy but not watery or thin. You may not need to add all 2 tablespoons (30 ml) of olive oil.

Form the falafel mixture into balls, about 2 inches (5 cm) in diameter. Lightly flatten them into patties with your hand and lay on the parchment-lined baking sheet. This recipe should make approximately eight to nine patties. Place the baking sheet in the oven and bake for 10 minutes. Carefully flip the patties over and bake for 6 to 8 minutes more. Remove the baking sheet from the oven and allow the falafel to cool slightly.

Place the hummus in a small bowl to serve alongside the falafel. Garnish with the diced cucumber and pomegranate arils.

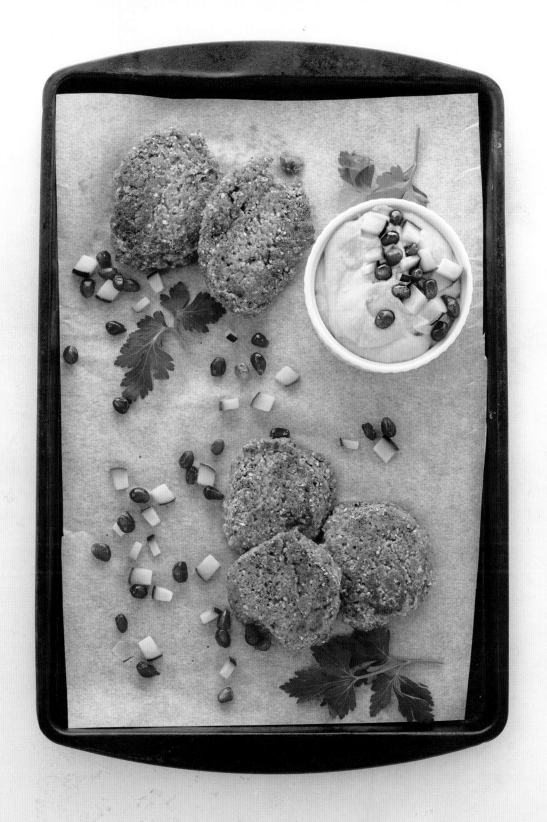

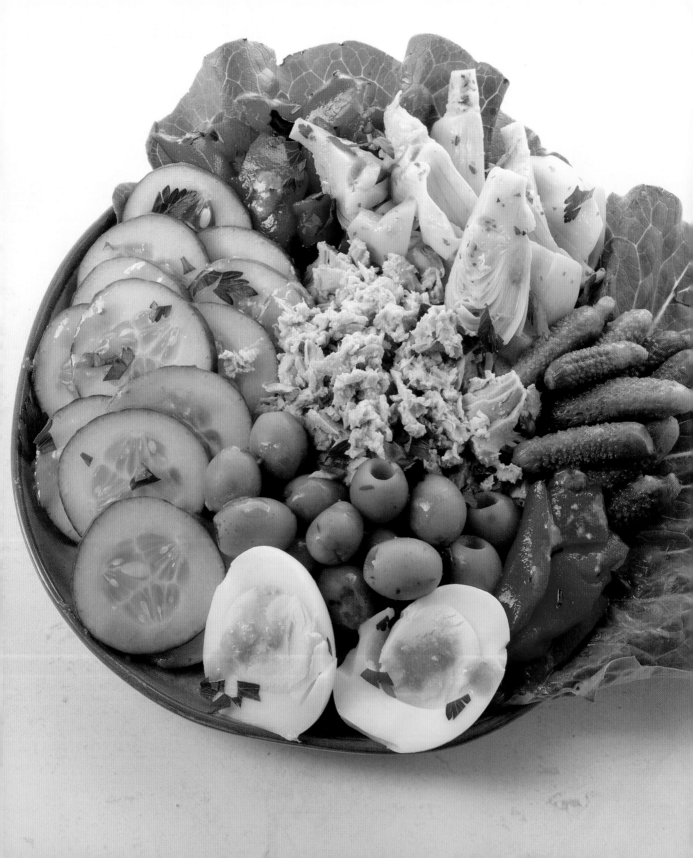

QUICK *and* VIBRANT NIÇOISE SALAD

MAKES 1 LARGE SALAD

Niçoise salads are one of my favorites because of all the great flavors and textures that go into them. This recipe takes the basic concept of this classic French salad and uses items that can be found in your pantry to create a zesty and crunchy, filling lunch that's also budget friendly.

My favorite part is the dressing—salty anchovies, rich olive oil and lots of garlic create the perfect vinaigrette. If you don't care for anchovies, you can simply omit them, but you may need to add a pinch of salt to the dressing in their place. If you are prepping this salad in advance and packing it up to take to work, I recommend keeping the dressing on the side until just before serving.

2 cloves garlic, minced

5–6 anchovy filets, drained

2 tbsp (30 ml) fresh lemon juice

¼ cup (60 ml) extra virgin olive oil

2 cups (94 g) roughly chopped romaine lettuce

½ medium cucumber, sliced

1 hard-boiled egg, cut in half

¼ cup (71 g) roasted red peppers, sliced

1 (2.7-oz [76-g]) can tuna, drained

½ cup (68 g) canned artichoke hearts, cut in half

¼ cup (54 g) olives

¼ cup (38 g) cornichons

In a food processor, combine the garlic, anchovy filets and lemon juice. Pulse until well chopped. Then with the food processor running, slowly add the olive oil. Puree the dressing until well combined and emulsified.

Combine the lettuce, cucumber, egg, roasted red peppers, tuna, artichoke hearts, olives and cornichons.

When ready to serve, pour the dressing over the top.

CRUNCHY BROCCOLI SALAD BOWL

MAKES 4 SERVINGS

A twist on the classic potluck dish, this broccoli salad recipe skips the heavy mayo. Instead, it features tangy Greek yogurt, giving this dish that same creamy texture but with a bit of protein and less saturated fat compared to mayo. The raisins and sunflower seeds offer wonderful texture. You can easily prepare this dish in advance and store the leftovers in the fridge for an easy, grab-on-the-go salad.

12 oz (340 g) broccoli florets

2 cups (220 g) shredded carrots

⅓ cup (48 g) golden raisins

¼ cup (34 g) sunflower seeds

¼ cup (40 g) diced red onion

1 cup (240 ml) plain Greek yogurt

1 clove garlic, minced

1 tsp fresh lemon juice

½ tsp white wine vinegar

¼ tsp salt, plus more to taste

¼ tsp pepper, plus more to taste

In a large bowl, combine the broccoli, carrots, raisins, sunflower seeds and onion. Set it aside.

In a small bowl or jar, combine the Greek yogurt, garlic, lemon juice, white wine vinegar, salt and pepper. Stir to combine and taste to see if additional salt or pepper needs to be added.

Pour the yogurt dressing over the bowl of broccoli salad. Mix well to combine. Serve immediately or refrigerate for up to 2 days.

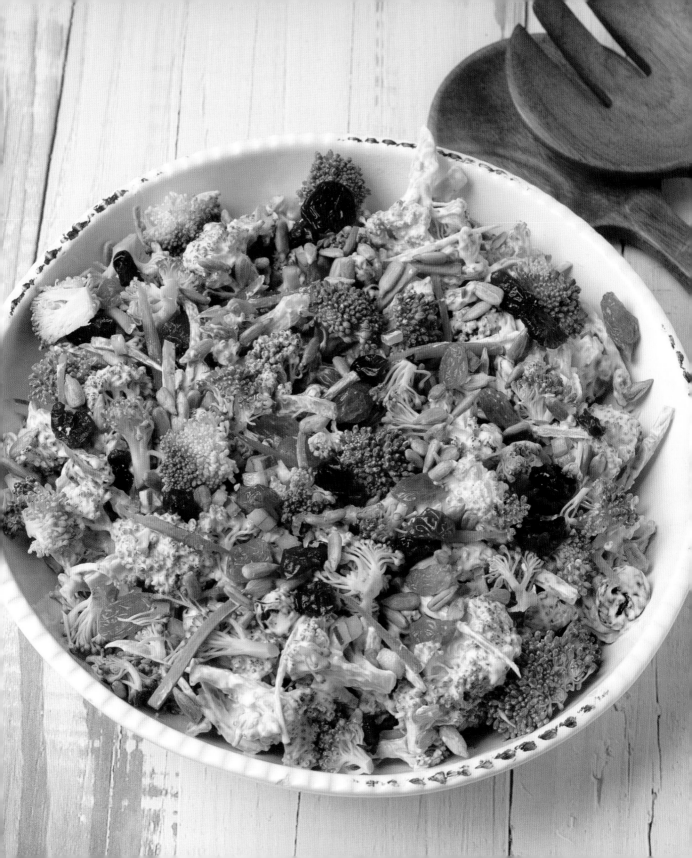

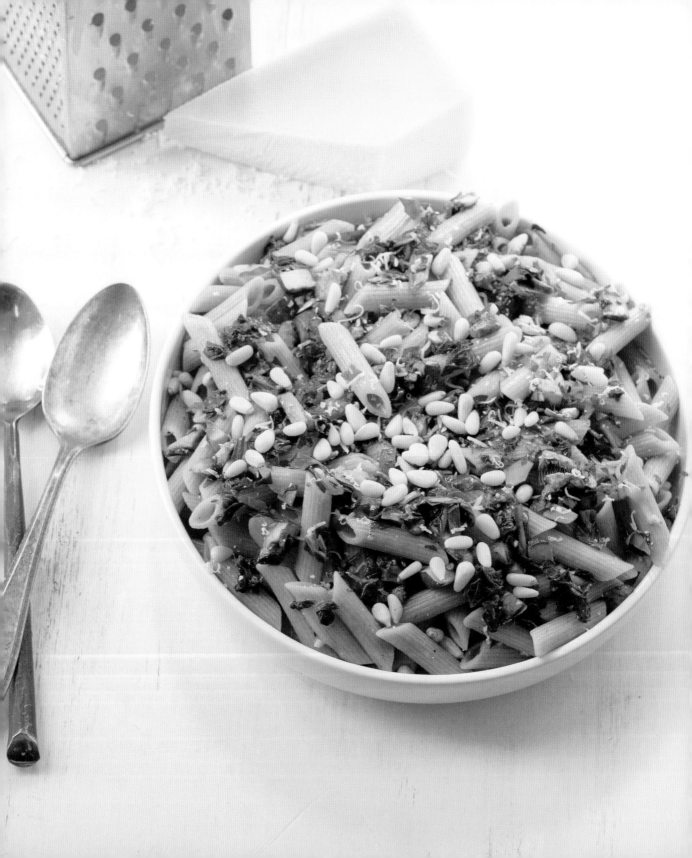

SPICY KALE PASTA *with* PINE NUTS

MAKES 4 SERVINGS

One of the things I remember most about eating pasta in Italy is the serving size compared to the giant bowls I was used to in the United States. The portions were smaller, but the flavor was off the charts.

This recipe uses whole wheat pasta and pairs it with hearty ingredients such as chopped mushrooms, leafy green kale and crunchy pine nuts. Instead of a cream-based sauce, the dish is lightly dressed with garlic, red pepper and a bit of Parmesan cheese to create a magnificent bowl of pasta bursting with bright flavors. I often serve this as a side dish for dinner and then set aside a small portion for lunch the following day.

16 oz (454 g) whole wheat pasta

2 tbsp (30 ml) extra virgin olive oil, divided

1 cup (80 g) chopped cremini mushrooms

4 cloves garlic, minced

2 cups (134 g) chopped baby kale

½ tsp salt

½ tsp red pepper flakes

¼ tsp pepper

¾ cup (75 g) grated Parmesan cheese

¼ cup (25 g) pine nuts

In a large pot, bring 6 cups (1.5 L) of water to a boil. Add the pasta and cook for 7 to 10 minutes. Be sure to reserve ½ cup (120 ml) of the pasta water before draining the pasta.

While the pasta is cooking, heat 1 tablespoon (15 ml) of the olive oil in a large skillet over medium heat. Add the mushrooms and garlic. Sauté for 2 minutes, stirring constantly to ensure the garlic doesn't burn.

Add the kale and ¼ cup (60 ml) of the reserved pasta water to the pan. Cook for 5 to 7 minutes and then stir in the salt, red pepper flakes and pepper. Remove the pan from the heat.

Once the pasta is drained, add it to the skillet with the kale. Stir to combine and add the Parmesan cheese. Add the remaining ¼ cup (60 ml) of reserved pasta water and stir everything together.

Serve in a large serving bowl, topped with the pine nuts.

BLACK BEAN–STUFFED SWEET POTATO *with* CHILI-LIME YOGURT

MAKES 2 SERVINGS

This sweet potato recipe is a hearty, healthy version of a traditional baked potato with all the toppings. Sweet potatoes offer a good dose of fiber, vitamins and minerals. This recipe adds even more flavor with filling black beans, creamy avocado and fresh herbs, all topped with a tangy, slightly spicy yogurt sauce.

2 medium sweet potatoes

1 (15.5-oz [439-g]) can black beans, drained and rinsed

¼ cup (60 ml) plain Greek yogurt

1 tbsp (3 g) chili powder

1 tbsp (15 ml) lime juice

1 medium avocado, diced

2 tbsp (2 g) chopped fresh cilantro

Start by positioning a rack in the center of the oven. Preheat the oven to 375°F (190°C, or gas mark 5).

Once the oven is warm, place the sweet potatoes directly on the center rack and bake for 45 minutes, or until cooked through and you can pierce with a fork. Allow them to cool slightly before stuffing.

While the sweet potatoes are cooking, place the black beans in a small saucepot. Heat over medium heat for 5 to 7 minutes. Remove the pot from the heat and set it aside.

In a small bowl, combine the Greek yogurt, chili powder and lime juice. Stir to combine and set it aside.

When the sweet potatoes are slightly cooled, cut a line down the center of each one to open them up. Fill each sweet potato with the cooked black beans, avocado and cilantro. Top each stuffed sweet potato with the yogurt sauce.

TIP: Sweet potatoes can be made in advance and reheated in the microwave, making them a great ingredient to add to your meal prep.

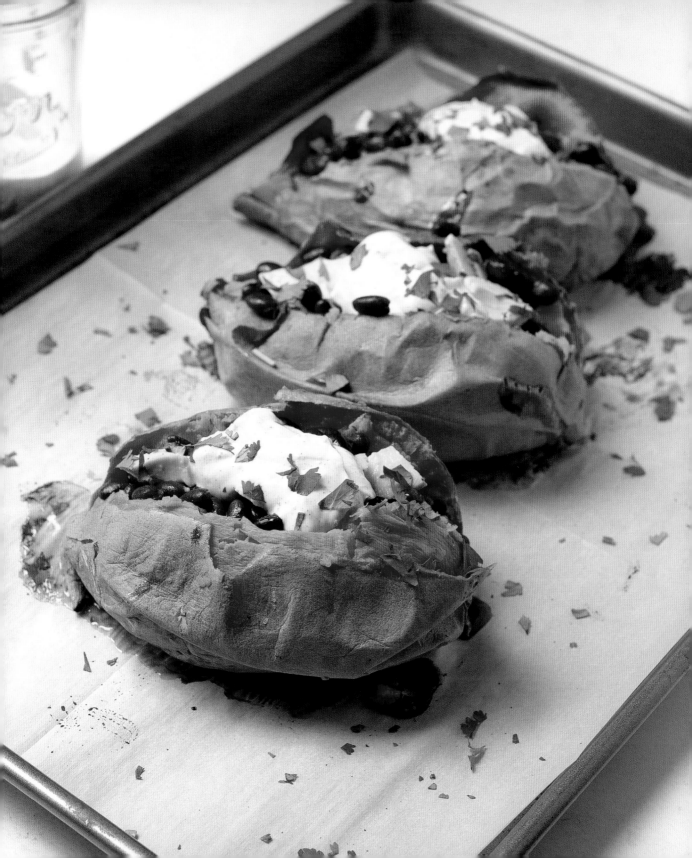

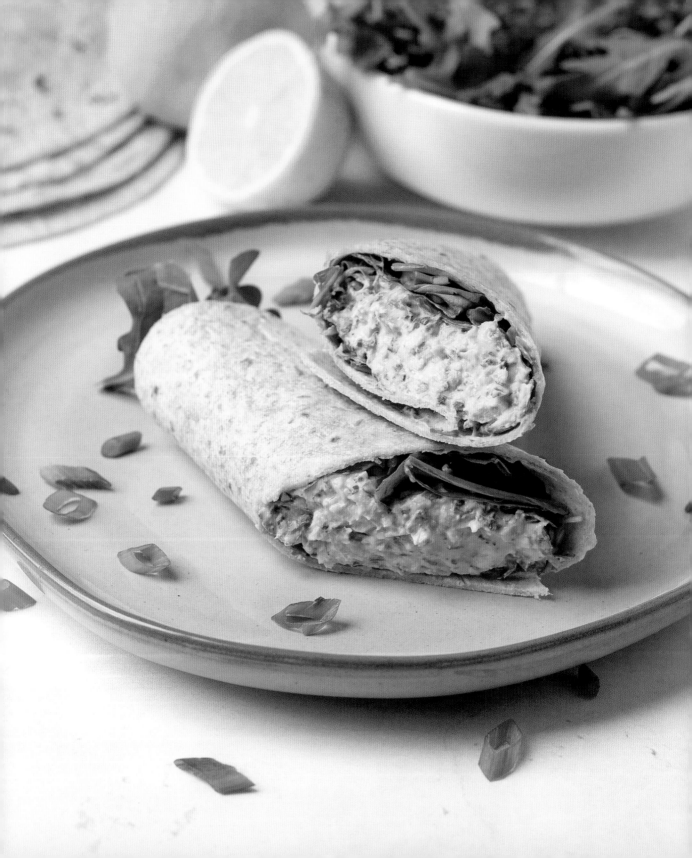

TANGY TUNA *and* ARUGULA WRAP

MAKES 2 WRAPS

This is one of my favorite lunch recipes. It's so simple, but tastes like it took a long list of ingredients to prepare. The tuna-and-yogurt mixture can be made in advance for easy weekday lunches. The tuna can also be changed out with shredded chicken—leftover rotisserie chicken works perfectly.

2 cups (68 g) arugula, divided

½ cup (30 g) chopped fresh Italian parsley

2 scallions, sliced

1 clove garlic, roughly chopped

1 cup (240 ml) plain Greek yogurt

1 tsp white wine vinegar

1 tsp fresh lemon juice

¼ tsp salt

¼ tsp pepper

8 oz (227 g) canned tuna, drained

2 whole wheat tortillas

In a food processor, combine 1 cup (34 g) of the arugula, the parsley, scallions, garlic, Greek yogurt, white wine vinegar, lemon juice, salt and pepper. Puree until well combined and the herbs are finely chopped. The mixture will be a bit chunky and that's perfect.

Pour the mixture into a mixing bowl and add the tuna. Mix until well combined.

To prepare the wrap, divide the remaining arugula and place it down the center of each tortilla. Spoon the tuna-and-yogurt mixture in the center of both tortillas. Wrap the tortillas and cut each one in half to serve.

SWEET *and* SAVORY APRICOT COUSCOUS SALAD

MAKES 4 SERVINGS

Couscous is one of my favorite grains to use because it cooks quickly and can be combined with so many different ingredients. To infuse even more flavor, I recommend cooking it in broth instead of plain water.

This sweet and savory salad features a touch of sweetness from dried fruit, crunch from slivered almonds and an easy oil-based vinaigrette that pulls it all together. The grilled chicken makes it a complete meal, but it would also work wonderfully served as a side dish. Trust me when I say you want to make a big enough batch to have leftovers the next day for lunch.

5 tbsp (75 ml) extra virgin olive oil

2 tbsp (30 ml) apple cider vinegar

½ tsp honey

¼ tsp salt

¼ tsp pepper

1 quart (960 ml) chicken broth

4 cups (690 g) whole wheat couscous, uncooked (If you can't find whole wheat, regular couscous is fine.)

2 (4-oz [113-g]) chicken breasts

4 scallions, sliced

1 cup (148 g) dried apricots

½ cup (54 g) sliced almonds

In a small bowl or jar, combine the olive oil, apple cider vinegar, honey, salt and pepper until well combined. Set it aside.

In a large pot, bring the chicken broth to a boil. Add the couscous, turn off the heat, cover and let stand for 5 to 8 minutes. Use a fork to fluff the couscous and allow it to cool slightly.

While the couscous cooks, grill the chicken breasts over medium heat for 4 to 5 minutes on each side. Once cooked through, remove the chicken from the grill and allow it to cool before slicing.

Add the couscous to a large bowl. Toss the couscous with half of the vinaigrette dressing. Then add the scallions, dried apricots and almonds. Gently toss to combine and taste. Add more vinaigrette as needed. Top the couscous with sliced, grilled chicken.

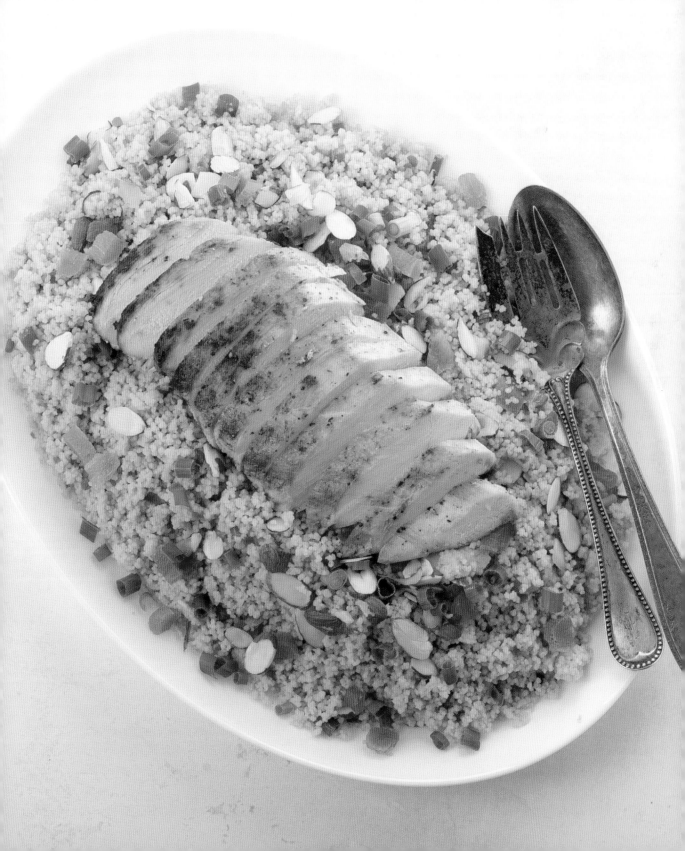

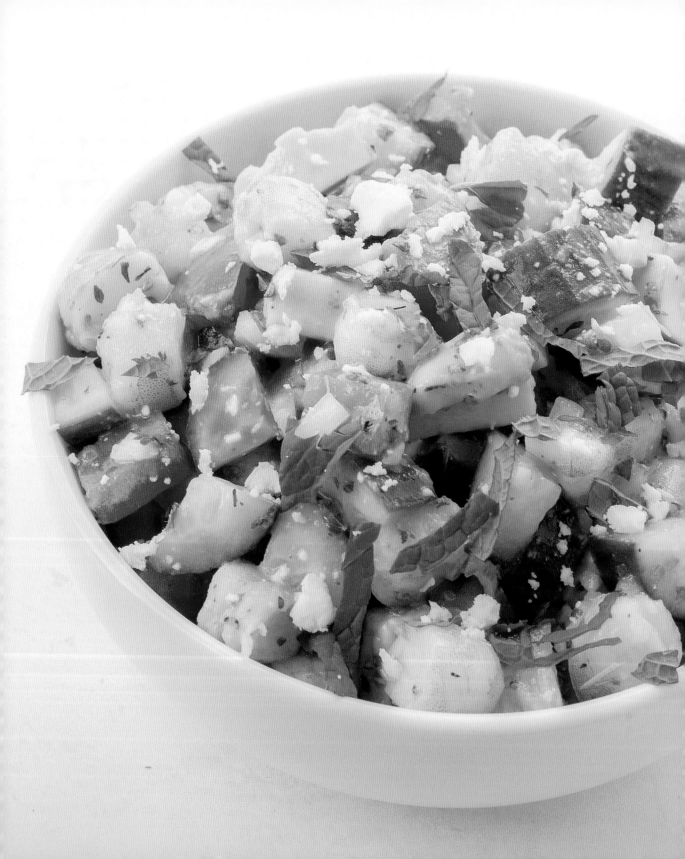

EFFORTLESS SHRIMP *and* AVOCADO BOWL

MAKES 2 SERVINGS

This no-cook shrimp bowl reminds me of ceviche, but without having to worry about "cooking" raw shrimp with lemon juice because this version is made with pre-cooked shrimp. It's tangy and bright with the fresh flavors of lime, lemon, oregano and mint to create an herby and citrusy lunch that comes together in minutes. This is the type of dish that you want to carve out time to just sit and enjoy. Even just twenty minutes during your weekday lunch break will make you appreciate all the fresh flavors that go into this dish. It really shows you what fresh, simple ingredients can do.

16 cooked jumbo shrimp, thawed, shelled and roughly chopped

1½ tbsp (23 ml) fresh lemon juice

2 tbsp (30 ml) extra virgin olive oil, divided

¼ tsp salt

¼ tsp pepper

1 tbsp (5 g) dried oregano

2 small Persian cucumbers, diced

1 Roma tomato, diced

½ avocado, diced

1 shallot, diced

2 tsp (10 ml) red wine vinegar

¼ cup (38 g) crumbled feta cheese

1 tbsp (6 g) chopped fresh mint

In a large bowl, combine the shrimp, lemon juice, 1 tablespoon (15 ml) of olive oil, salt, pepper and oregano. Allow the shrimp to marinate slightly while you chop and prepare the other ingredients.

When ready, add the cucumbers, tomato, avocado, shallot, remaining olive oil and red wine vinegar to the bowl with the shrimp. Stir to combine.

When ready to serve, top the shrimp bowl with the feta cheese and mint.

HERB-*and*-GARLIC CHICKEN SOUVLAKI SALAD

MAKES 2 SERVINGS

When I was in Greece, I ate some form of chicken souvlaki at least once a day. I just couldn't get enough of the juicy, grilled chicken that had been marinated in fresh herbs and combined with tangy yogurt sauce, red onion and tomato. This recipe is a play on the chicken souvlaki gyro, just a bit deconstructed. You get all the same great flavors, packed with even more veggies because it's served as a salad rather than in a pita.

It's best to marinate the chicken for at least 30 minutes before cooking. I prefer to leave it in the marinade overnight to really get all those flavors into the chicken. You could also precook the chicken, making it easier to bring for on-the-go lunches.

1 lb (454 g) chicken breast tenders

4 cloves garlic, minced

2 tbsp (30 ml) extra virgin olive oil

1 tbsp (5 g) dried oregano

½ tsp salt

½ tsp pepper

1 tbsp (15 ml) fresh lemon juice

1 cup (100 g) cherry tomatoes, halved

1 medium cucumber, diced

¼ cup (40 g) diced red onion

¼ cup (54 g) olives

¼ cup (15 g) chopped fresh Italian parsley

¼ cup (60 ml) Traditional Tzatziki Sauce with Fresh Dill (page 166)

Place the chicken in a large resealable bag or a glass dish. Add the garlic, olive oil, oregano, salt, pepper and lemon juice. Toss to coat the chicken with the oil and spices. Allow it to marinate for at least 30 minutes or overnight.

While the chicken is marinating, divide the tomatoes, cucumber, onion and olives equally between two large plates or bowls.

Once the chicken has marinated, sauté it in a skillet over medium heat for 4 to 5 minutes on each side. Remove the chicken from the heat and allow it to cool slightly before dicing.

Divide the cooked chicken between the two plates. Garnish with parsley and serve with tzatziki sauce.

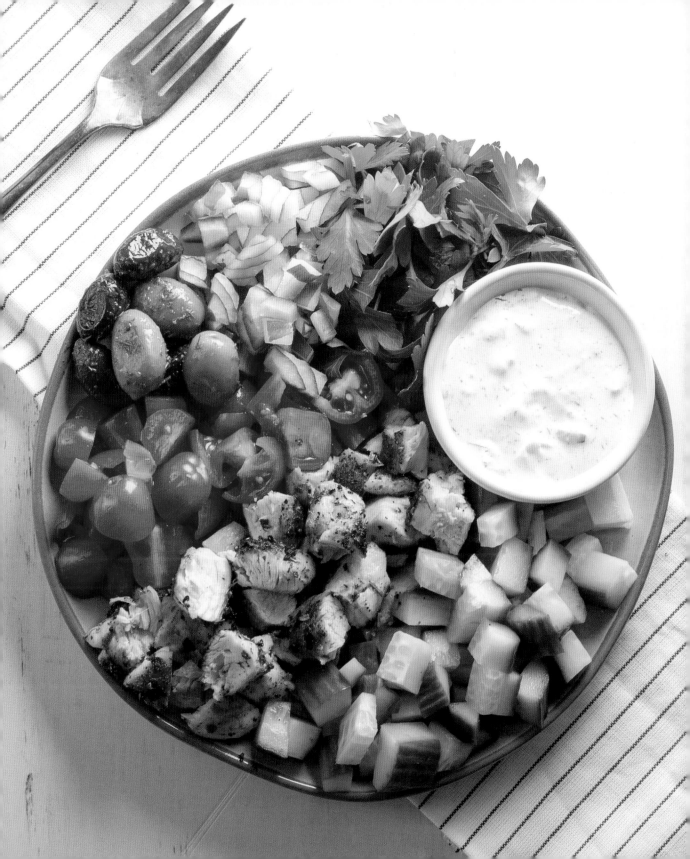

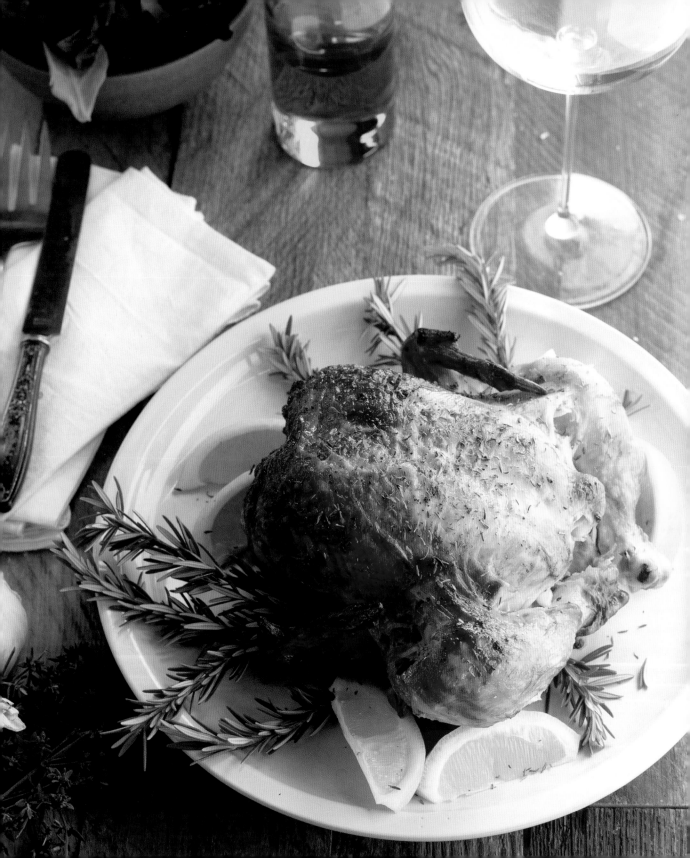

Wholesome DINNERS

Unlike other diets that are very restrictive and involve eliminating certain food groups, counting calories or eating at set times, the Mediterranean diet is actually quite easy to adapt to your current lifestyle. There are no black-and-white rules. It's also very family friendly because you can use ingredients, foods and recipes that you already eat and enjoy. In my opinion, any dish can be changed slightly to fit into the Mediterranean diet, it doesn't have to be a "Mediterranean" recipe.

A good place to start is by looking at a meal you would normally eat. See how you could change it a little to meet more of the Mediterranean diet guidelines. Let's say you enjoy spaghetti with meatballs. You could use whole wheat pasta in place of regular pasta, add mushrooms, bell peppers and spinach to your spaghetti sauce, and use ground turkey meatballs in place of beef meatballs. Those simple, Mediterranean diet–inspired changes incorporate more whole grains and vegetables into your dinner, as well as reducing red meat.

Dinner is also a great time to sit down and enjoy a meal with others, whether it be family, friends, coworkers or a neighbor. A big part of the Mediterranean lifestyle is taking the time to slow down and connect with others while celebrating good food. While that isn't always possible with today's hectic schedules, it's important to try and find the balance between quick weeknight dinners and meals where you have a bit more time.

The dinners in this chapter include quick weeknight meals that are tasty without being overly time consuming, such as the Baked Cod with Broccolini Amandine (page 84). Other recipes take more time and are meant to be enjoyed in a relaxed setting, such as the Braised Chicken Cacciatore (page 112).

All of the recipes are made with delicious ingredients designed to help you incorporate more vegetables, whole grains, beans, legumes, nuts, seeds, fresh herbs and spices into your everyday life. My biggest advice is to try and make plants the star of your meals and use other ingredients in smaller amounts to complement those fruits, vegetables and whole grains.

I also recommend making extra batches of dinners you love and saving the leftovers for lunch or freezing them for later use. The Lemon and Caper Chicken Piccata Meatballs (page 100) make the most amazing weekday lunch, so I always make sure to double that recipe.

BAKED COD *with* BROCCOLINI AMANDINE

Makes 2 servings

This is the perfect fish recipe because it's so easy and comes together quickly. The fish is flaky and the crispy breadcrumb topping is seasoned beautifully with dried herbs and garlic. While the fish bakes in the oven, the broccolini gets lightly sautéed and then topped with toasted almonds to create a fresh, vibrant dish that's ready in under 20 minutes. If you can't find broccolini, use broccoli florets or green beans instead.

½ cup (25 g) panko-style breadcrumbs

2 tbsp (30 ml) extra virgin olive oil, divided

1 tsp garlic powder

1 tsp dried parsley

¼ tsp salt

¼ tsp pepper

2 (6-oz [170-g]) cod filets

8 oz (227 g) broccolini

½ cup (54 g) slivered almonds

1 tbsp (15 ml) fresh lemon juice

Start by positioning a rack in the center of the oven. Preheat the oven to 425°F (220°C, or gas mark 6). Line a rimmed baking sheet with parchment paper.

In a small bowl, combine the breadcrumbs, 1 tablespoon (15 ml) of the olive oil, the garlic powder, parsley, salt and pepper. Mix the ingredients together until well combined.

Place the cod filets on the baking sheet. Use a spoon to evenly press the breadcrumb mixture on top of the cod filets. Press down lightly with the spoon to help the breadcrumb mixture stick to the fish. Place the baking sheet on the center rack of the oven and bake for 15 minutes. You'll know the fish is done when you can easily flake off a piece with a fork.

Line a dish with a paper towel. While the fish is cooking, bring 6 cups (1.5 L) of water to a boil in a large pot. Once boiling, quickly place the broccolini in the water to blanch. Remove the broccolini with tongs after 3 minutes in the water and set it on the lined dish to drain slightly.

In a medium skillet, heat the remaining olive oil over medium heat. Add the blanched broccolini and sauté for 5 to 8 minutes, until slightly softened. Add the almonds and sauté for 2 minutes, stirring constantly.

Place the baked cod and broccolini-almond mixture on two plates and drizzle with the lemon juice.

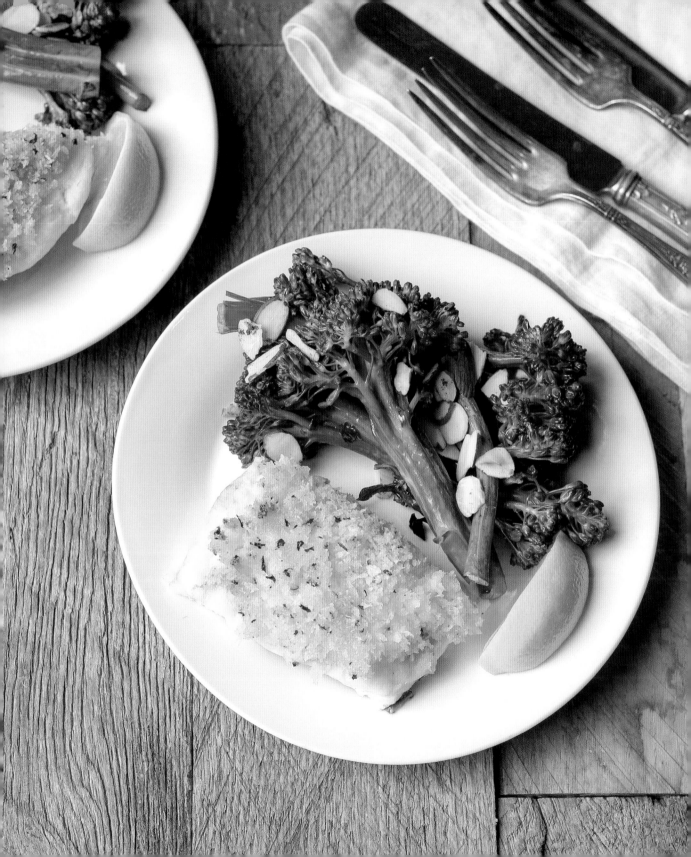

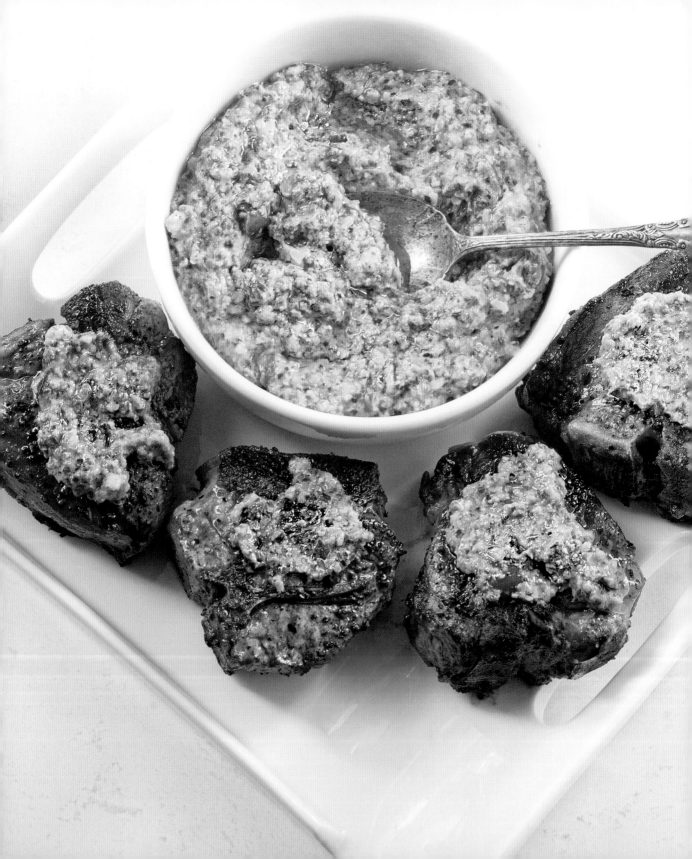

GRILLED LAMB *with* PISTACHIO-OLIVE TAPENADE

MAKES 4 SERVINGS

This dinner is a showstopper, so I love making it for dinner parties because everyone thinks you spent all day making it. However, lamb is so quick to grill that it's perfect for any night of the week. The pistachio-olive tapenade is just bursting with fresh herbs, garlic, olives and citrus. You can adjust the heat-level by increasing the red pepper flakes if you like a bit more spice, but I've found this amount to be the perfect little kick. I like to make extra and keep it in the fridge to put on scrambled eggs, baked chicken or roasted vegetables.

The beauty of lamb is that the flavor is so concentrated that you don't need a big serving to feel full and satisfied. It is considered red meat, so I recommend enjoying it in moderation and savoring each and every bite.

1 lb (454 g) lamb loin chops

½ tsp salt

½ tsp pepper

1 large shallot, roughly chopped

1 clove garlic, roughly chopped

1 cup (60 g) chopped fresh Italian parsley

⅓ cup (31 g) chopped fresh mint

½ cup (62 g) pistachios, shells removed

2 tbsp (30 ml) fresh lemon juice

¼ cup (54 g) olives, pitted

1 tbsp (7 g) capers

1 tsp red pepper flakes

½ cup (120 ml) extra virgin olive oil

Allow your lamb loin chops to come to room temperature, then evenly sprinkle them with the salt and pepper. Heat a grill pan or heavy-duty skillet over medium-high heat.

While the lamb is coming to temperature, make the tapenade. In a food processor, combine the shallot, garlic, parsley, mint, pistachios, lemon juice, olives, capers and red pepper flakes. Pulse everything until finely chopped. With the food processor running, slowly add in the olive oil. Puree the tapenade until well combined and similar to the consistency of a thick pesto. Set aside.

Grill your lamb for 4 to 5 minutes on each side. You can tell your lamb is done by pressing lightly into the surface. If it gives easily but is still firm to the touch, it is done and cooked to medium-rare. If you prefer your lamb more well done, cook until the texture when pressed is more firm with little to no give. Remove from the heat and allow to rest for 5 to 8 minutes. Serve with the prepared tapenade.

ONE-PAN LEMON *and* ARTICHOKE BAKED CHICKEN

MAKES 4 SERVINGS

If you and your family need a relaxed, delicious, homemade meal that doesn't take a lot of effort to bring to the table, this is the recipe for you. This entire meal is cooked in a single pan and is just bursting with the bright flavors of lemon and artichokes. It also uses canned artichoke hearts, making it perfect for any season and very budget friendly.

To add even more veggies to this meal, serve the chicken with the Crunchy Chickpea Salad with Fresh Herbs (page 131) or a warm bowl of Creamy Spinach and Cauliflower Soup with Spiced Chickpeas (page 143). And be sure to add a slice of Homemade Garlic and Herb Flatbread (page 45) to soak up all those lemony cooking juices in the bottom of the pan.

1 lb (454 g) boneless, skinless chicken thighs

2 tbsp (30 ml) extra virgin olive oil, divided

3 tbsp (20 g) Greek Seasoning Spice Blend (page 177), divided

1 (14.1-oz [400-g]) can artichoke hearts, cut in half

1 lemon, sliced

⅓ cup (72 g) olives

Marinate the chicken thighs in a resealable bag or a glass dish with 1 tablespoon (15 ml) of olive oil and 2 tablespoons (14 g) of Greek seasoning for at least 30 minutes. If you have the time, the chicken can be marinated for up to 24 hours before making this dish.

While the chicken is marinating, preheat the oven to 350°F (175°C, or gas mark 4). Once the chicken is ready, place it in an ovenproof baking dish or skillet. Add the artichoke hearts, lemon and olives to the dish by simply placing them around the chicken thighs. Sprinkle the remaining Greek seasoning over the top of the entire dish.

Cover the baking dish with foil and place it in the oven for 12 minutes. Remove the foil and bake for 10 to 12 minutes, or until the chicken is cooked through and golden brown.

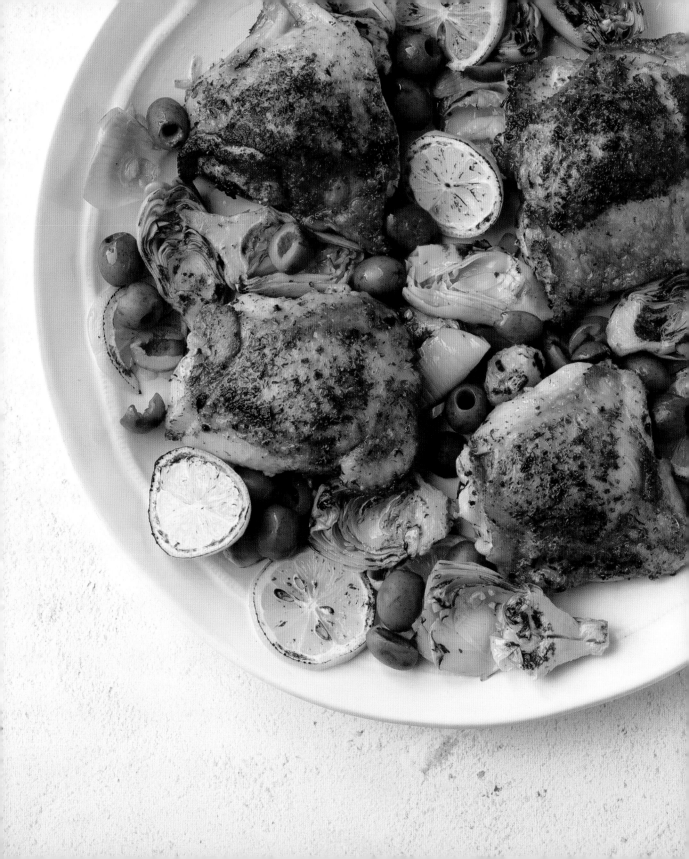

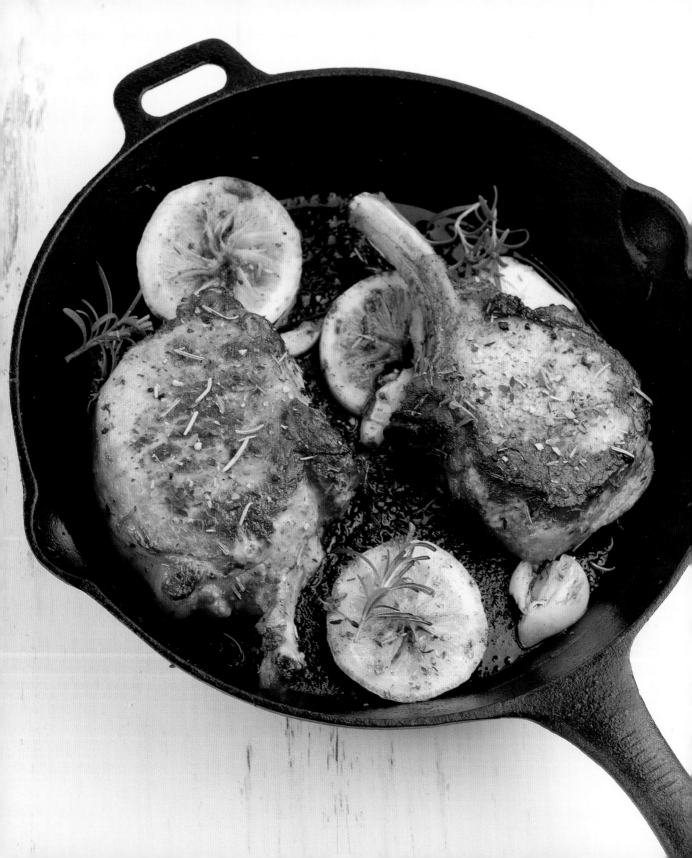

SIMPLE HERB-MARINATED PORK CHOPS

MAKES 2 SERVINGS

The key to these simple pork chops is the herb-and-garlic marinade. It infuses such an amazing and rich flavor that you'll be scraping your plate for more—no heavy cream sauces needed. This is a favorite at my house and makes great leftovers for lunch the next day.

If you can't find bone-in pork loin chops, you could use pork tenderloin or boneless pork chops instead. The cooking time will increase for a whole tenderloin, but will decrease if you use boneless chops.

1 lemon

2 (21-oz [595-g]) bone-in pork loin chops

¼ cup (60 ml) plus 1 tbsp (15 ml) extra virgin olive oil, divided

3 cloves garlic, crushed

2 tbsp (7 g) dried rosemary

Cut the lemon in half and juice one half. Cut the second half into slices. In a resealable bag or a large dish, place the pork loin chops on the bottom. Cover them with ¼ cup (60 ml) of olive oil, the lemon juice and slices, garlic and rosemary. Shake or stir to combine, ensuring that the entire surface of the pork chops is covered with the marinade.

Place the pork chops in the fridge for at least 30 minutes or up to 24 hours.

Once ready to cook, heat the remaining 1 tablespoon (15 ml) olive oil in a large skillet over medium heat. Once the oil is warm, add the pork chops and the remaining marinade from the bag to the skillet and cook for 8 minutes on each side.

TIP: Pair this dish with a flavorful side, such as the Fresh Lemon and Herb Tabbouleh Salad (page 123) or Warm French Lentil Salad with Dijon (page 127), for a complete meal.

FLAVORFUL TURKEY *and* WHITE BEAN SOUP

MAKES 4 SERVINGS

This soup is so hearty and filling that it makes a complete meal in a single bowl. The tender ground turkey and the creamy cannellini beans leave you feeling nourished while offering up some protein and fiber. Fresh rosemary and dried thyme give the stock a wonderful flavor, and the earthy spinach and kale wilt into the warm, simmered soup to create even more texture and a beautiful pop of color.

This soup makes great leftovers as it reheats nicely, making it an excellent weekday lunch option.

1 tbsp (15 ml) extra virgin olive oil

1 lb (454 g) ground turkey

2 carrots, peeled and sliced

1 medium onion, diced

3 cloves garlic, minced

3 sprigs fresh rosemary

1 tsp dried thyme

½ tsp salt

¼ tsp pepper

1 (15.5-oz [439-g]) can cannellini beans, drained and rinsed

1 quart (960 ml) chicken broth

1 cup (30 g) spinach

1 cup (67 g) chopped kale

In a large stockpot, heat the olive oil over medium heat. Once warm, add the ground turkey and sauté until lightly browned, about 4 to 6 minutes. Add the carrots, onion and garlic to the pot. Sauté until the vegetables are soft, about 6 minutes.

Add the rosemary, thyme, salt, pepper, cannellini beans and chicken broth. Stir the mixture together and bring it to a boil. Once boiling, reduce the heat to low and simmer for 20 minutes.

Remove the sprigs of rosemary, and add the spinach and kale leaves. Stir to combine and ladle the soup into bowls.

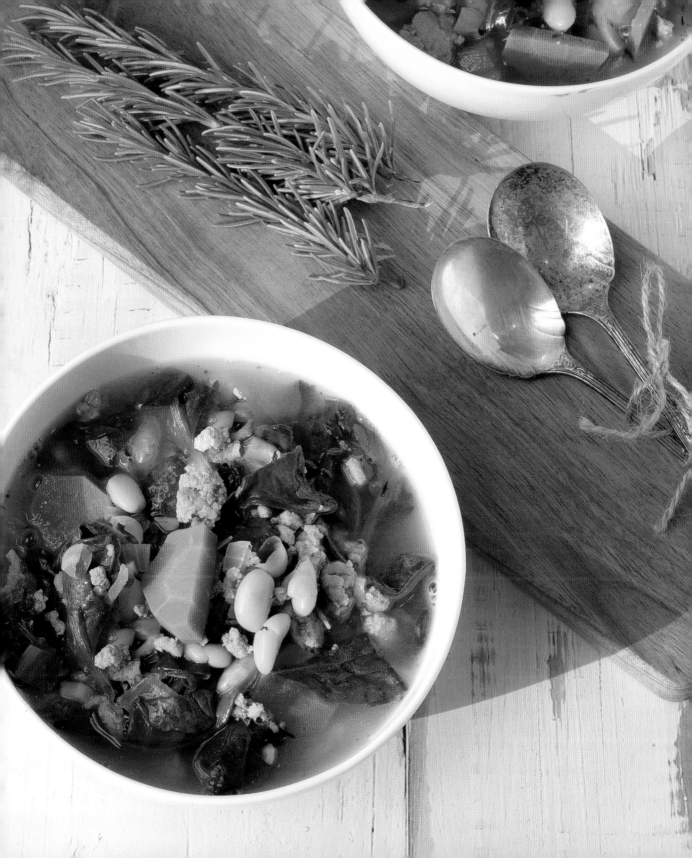

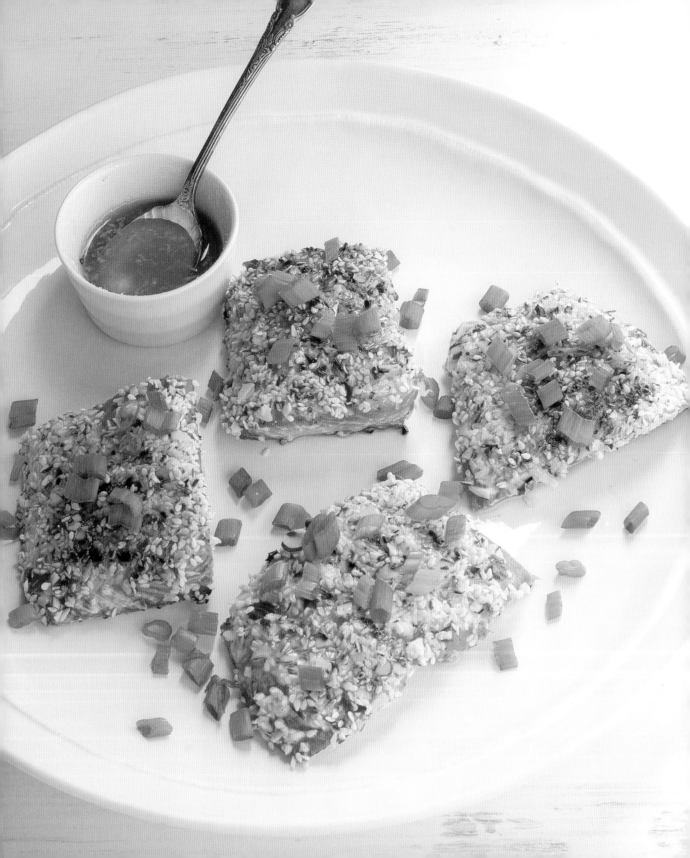

ALMOND *and* SESAME—CRUSTED SALMON

MAKES 4 SERVINGS

This salmon dish is a delicious and easy way to get your recommended weekly serving of fish. It's flaky and tender, and it has a fantastic almond and sesame flavor. A simple sauce finishes it off without being too sweet or overpowering. If you are new to eating fish, this is a great "starter" recipe because it only takes 10 minutes to cook and salmon is generally mild in flavor.

⅓ cup (48 g) finely chopped almonds

3 tbsp (27 g) sesame seeds

4 (4-oz [113-g]) salmon filets

3 tbsp (45 ml) extra virgin olive oil, divided

1 tbsp (15 ml) honey

1 clove garlic, minced

2 scallions, green part only, sliced

Place the almonds and sesame seeds on a shallow plate and lightly stir to combine.

Brush the tops of the salmon filets with 1 tablespoon (15 ml) of the olive oil and press the top lightly into the plate of almonds and sesame seeds. Ensure the top of each salmon filet is evenly coated with the mixture.

Heat 1 tablespoon (15 ml) of the olive oil in a large skillet over medium heat. Press the salmon filets, almond crust side down, in the skillet and sear for 4 minutes. Carefully flip the filets over and cook for 5 minutes.

While the salmon is cooking, combine the remaining 1 tablespoon (15 ml) of olive oil, honey and garlic in a small bowl.

When the salmon is done cooking, brush the top of each filet with a teaspoon of the honey dressing. Garnish the top of each filet with the scallion greens.

TIP: You can tell the salmon is done when the fish is no longer raw/red in color. Be sure it has turned pink and the fish flakes off easily with a fork.

BAKED QUINOA-STUFFED PEPPERS

Makes 4 servings

Stuffed bell peppers were a classic dish at my house growing up. My mom used to make them with ground beef, tomatoes and rice. I've put a little Mediterranean spin on her recipe by stuffing these bell peppers with fluffy quinoa, hearty lentils and fresh herbs. The entire dish is then drizzled with a delightfully tangy tahini dressing.

This is one of the first vegetarian dishes that I served to my husband that he completely devoured. It wasn't until I told him that it was vegetarian that he even noticed there wasn't any meat.

1 cup (168 g) quinoa

4 bell peppers, assorted colors

1 cup (200 g) cooked lentils

1 tsp extra virgin olive oil

1 clove garlic, minced

½ shallot, diced

1 (14.5-oz [411-g]) can fire-roasted tomatoes, drained

1 tbsp (4 g) chopped fresh Italian parsley

2 tbsp (30 ml) Extra Creamy Tahini Dressing (page 174)

Start by preheating the oven to 400°F (200°C, or gas mark 6). Cook the quinoa according to the package directions.

Slice all 4 bell peppers in half lengthwise and then remove any seeds and membrane. Place the sliced bell peppers face up in a large baking dish and set it aside.

In a medium bowl, combine the cooked quinoa and lentils. Set it aside.

In a small pan, heat the olive oil over medium heat. Once warm, add the garlic and shallot and sauté for 1 to 2 minutes. Add the mixture to the bowl with the lentils and quinoa. Add the tomatoes and parsley. Mix well.

Spoon the lentil mixture into each of the bell peppers in your baking dish. The bell peppers should be overflowing with the lentil-quinoa mixture. Place the baking dish in the oven and bake for 15 to 20 minutes.

Just before serving, drizzle the top of each stuffed bell pepper with the creamy tahini dressing.

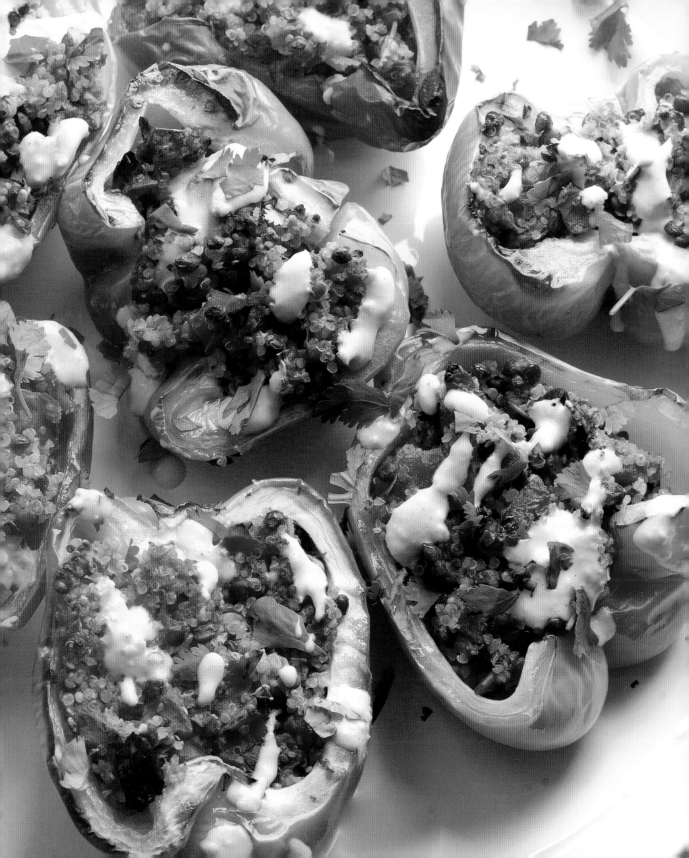

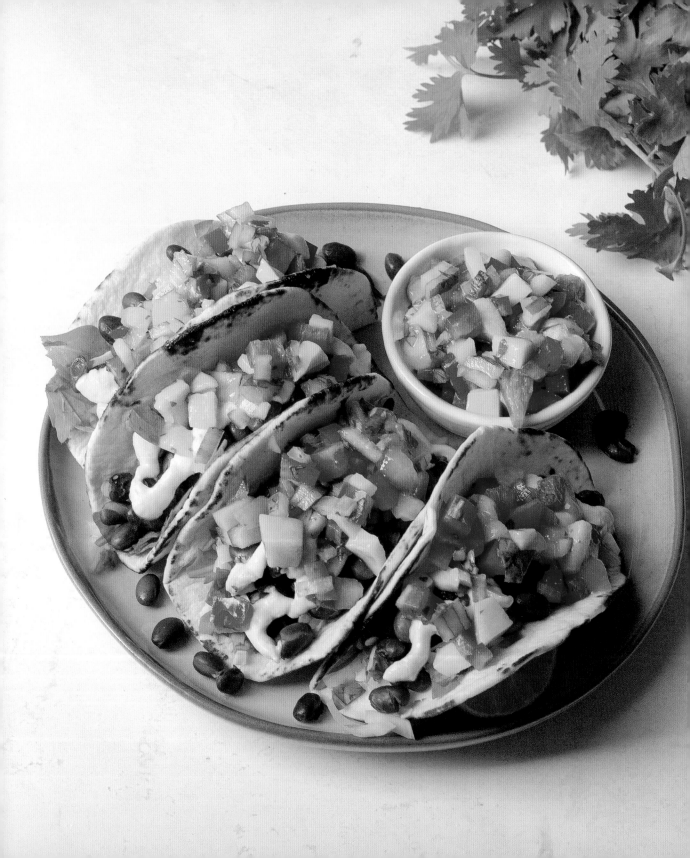

MANGO *and* BLACK BEAN TACOS *with* AVOCADO YOGURT

MAKES 8 TACOS

This recipe is a great example of how to apply the principles of the Mediterranean diet to recipes that don't exactly seem like they would fit . . . like tacos. These plant-based tacos are full of fiber-filled black beans and the fresh flavors of juicy mango, spicy jalapeno and crunchy bell peppers. It's all topped with bright lime juice and a creamy avocado yogurt that's made in minutes.

2 cups (330 g) chopped mango (If using frozen, thaw before use in a colander.)

½ medium red onion, finely diced

1 medium bell pepper, diced

1 small jalapeño, seeds removed and diced

2 tbsp (30 ml) lime juice, divided

½ cup (8 g) chopped fresh cilantro

1 (15.5-oz [439-g]) can black beans, drained and rinsed

1 avocado, pitted and peeled

1 cup (240 ml) plain Greek yogurt

¼ tsp salt

¼ tsp pepper

1 cup (30 g) finely chopped lettuce

8 small flour or corn tortillas, lightly charred

Make the mango salsa first so that it has time to marinate while the rest of the dish comes together. In a small bowl, combine the mango, onion, bell pepper, jalapeño, 1 tablespoon (15 ml) of the lime juice and the cilantro. Stir well to combine it all together and set it aside.

In a small pot over medium heat, cook the black beans for 3 to 5 minutes. Remove the pot from the heat and allow it to cool slightly.

In another small bowl, smash the avocado with the back of a fork and then stir in the Greek yogurt, remaining lime juice, salt and pepper. Stir well to combine.

To assemble the tacos, place lettuce in the bottom of each tortilla. Top with the black beans and some of the avocado yogurt, and finish with the mango salsa.

TIP: In place of mango, you could use pineapple, strawberries or even kiwi.

LEMON *and* CAPER CHICKEN PICCATA MEATBALLS

MAKES 14 MEATBALLS

This recipe takes all those amazing flavors of traditional chicken piccata and presents them in meatball form. Tender and juicy ground chicken meatballs simmer in a vibrant sauce with lemon, a splash of white wine, plenty of garlic, salty capers and a bit of turmeric for flavor and color. The end result is a bright, flavor-packed dish that is perfect with whole wheat pasta, potatoes or even served as an appetizer.

MEATBALLS

1 lb (454 g) ground chicken

⅓ cup (33 g) grated Parmesan cheese

3 cloves garlic, minced

1 tbsp (1 g) lemon zest

⅔ cup (39 g) panko-style breadcrumbs

½ tsp salt

¼ tsp pepper

1 tbsp (4 g) chopped fresh Italian parsley

1 large egg

1 tbsp (15 ml) extra virgin olive oil

SAUCE

2 tbsp (30 ml) extra virgin olive oil

1 tbsp (8 g) all-purpose flour

½ cup (120 ml) chicken broth

¼ cup (60 ml) fresh lemon juice

⅓ cup (80 ml) white wine

2 cloves garlic, minced

1 tbsp (5 g) ground turmeric

1 tbsp (7 g) capers

To make the chicken meatballs: In a large bowl, combine the chicken, Parmesan cheese, garlic, lemon zest, breadcrumbs, salt, pepper, parsley and egg. Using your hands, mix until everything is just combined. Be sure not to overmix.

Form the chicken mixture into tablespoon-sized (60-g) meatballs. I like to use a small scoop or a tablespoon to ensure they are all the same size. This will create approximately 14 meatballs.

Heat the olive oil in a large skillet over medium-high heat. Add the meatballs to the pan; don't overcrowd the pan, and cook in batches if you need to. Cook for about 3 minutes on each side. Once the meatballs are lightly browned on each side, remove the meatballs from the skillet and place them on a large plate.

To make the sauce: Add the olive oil to the same skillet. Whisk in the flour and continue to whisk until a thick roux forms. Slowly add in the chicken broth, lemon juice and white wine. Whisk until combined and then add the garlic, turmeric and capers. Whisk quickly to combine and then add the chicken meatballs back to the pan. Allow the meatballs to finish cooking in the sauce for 2 to 3 minutes before serving.

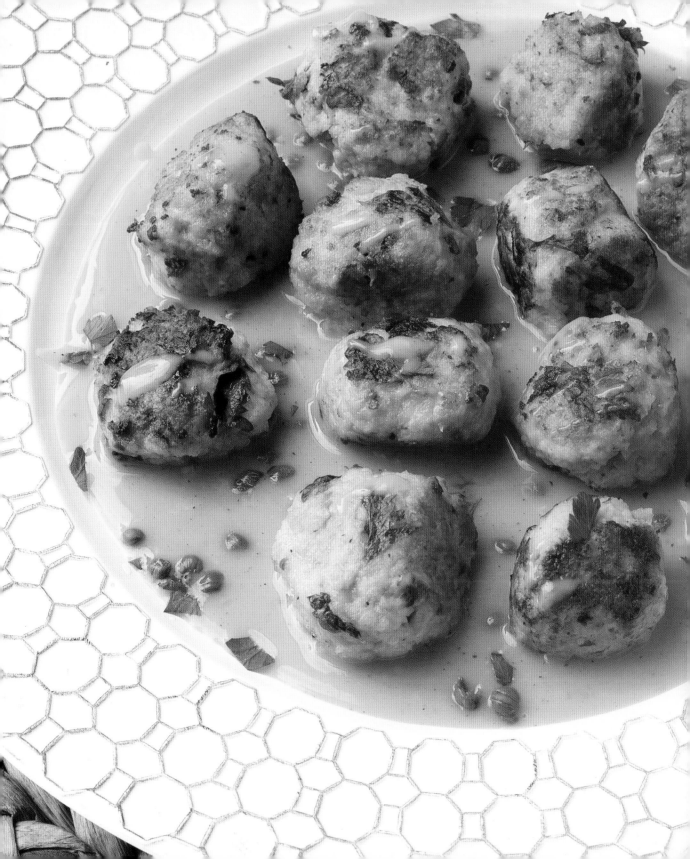

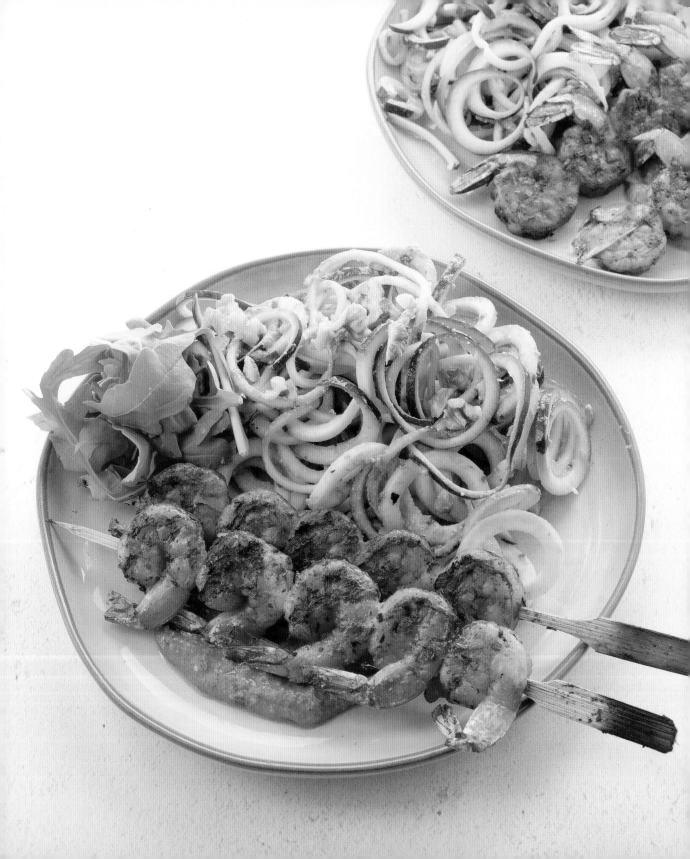

QUICK GRILLED SHRIMP *with* PESTO *and* ZUCCHINI NOODLES

MAKES 4 SERVINGS

This is a perfect weeknight meal that will wow your taste buds but won't take too much time to prepare. You could make the prep time even shorter by spiralizing your zucchini noodles in advance; in a pinch, many large chain grocery stores sell pre-spiralized zucchini in the produce section. If you haven't had zucchini noodles, they are a great way to add more vegetables to your diet. I think they are a fun and tasty alternative to regular pasta. The consistency is a bit crisper than regular noodles, so another option if you are new to zoodles is to substitute half the zucchini noodles with spaghetti or fettuccine.

20 raw shrimp, tails and shells removed

2 tbsp (30 ml) extra virgin olive oil, divided

1 clove garlic, minced

1 tbsp (5 g) smoked paprika

¼ tsp salt

¼ tsp pepper

3 medium zucchini

¼ cup (56 g) Peppery Arugula-Walnut Pesto (page 173)

Chopped walnuts and chopped arugula, for garnish (optional)

In a large resealable bag or a glass dish, combine the shrimp, 1 tablespoon (15 ml) of olive oil, garlic, paprika, salt and pepper. Set it aside.

While the shrimp are marinating, use a spiralizer to create zucchini noodles. If you don't have a spiralizer, you can simply slice the zucchini into long, thin, noodle-like slices.

Heat a large skillet over medium heat and add the remaining olive oil. Once warm, add the spiralized zucchini and lightly sauté for 2 to 3 minutes, just until the zucchini softens slightly. Remove the skillet from the heat and pour the sautéed zucchini into a large bowl. Lightly toss the zucchini noodles with the pesto.

Using a wooden or metal skewer, thread 5 shrimp onto each skewer. Once the shrimp skewers are assembled, grill them on a grill pan over medium-high heat. They cook quickly, so you only need to grill for about 2 minutes on each side. If you don't have a grill pan, you can also sauté the skewers in a pan over medium-high heat.

Once the shrimp are fully cooked, serve them on a plate with the pesto zucchini noodles. Garnish with walnuts and arugula, if desired.

TIP: If you are using wooden skewers, soak them in water for about 5 to 10 minutes before using. This will help prevent any wood from splintering off or burning while cooking.

JUICY LAMB *and* MUSHROOM BURGERS

MAKES 4 BURGERS

Lamb burgers are extremely popular in Greece, and this recipe uses roasted mushrooms to replace some of the ground lamb in the dish. It's a great way to add extra flavor and keep the heartiness of the dish without having to use as much red meat. To create some variety, you could easily substitute ground beef, turkey or chicken for these burgers.

8 oz (227 g) cremini mushrooms, chopped

2 tbsp (30 ml) extra virgin olive oil, divided

¼ tsp salt

¼ tsp pepper

1 lb (454 g) ground lamb

2 tbsp (8 g) finely chopped fresh Italian parsley

1 large egg

¼ cup (60 ml) Traditional Tzatziki Sauce with Fresh Dill (page 166)

4 hamburger buns

1 small red onion, thinly sliced into rings

1 cup (34 g) arugula

Preheat the oven to 400°F (200°C, or gas mark 6). Line a large baking sheet with parchment paper.

Spread the mushrooms in a single layer on the parchment-lined baking sheet. Drizzle them with 1 tablespoon (15 ml) of the olive oil and sprinkle with the salt and pepper. Place the baking sheet in the oven and roast for 20 minutes. Remove the baking sheet and allow the mushrooms to cool slightly.

In a large bowl, combine the ground lamb, parsley, egg and the cooled mushrooms. Use your hands to combine the mixture until everything is well mixed. Form into four equal-sized patties.

Heat a large grill pan or skillet over medium-high heat. Add the remaining olive oil. Place the lamb burgers on the grill pan and cook them for 4 minutes on each side for a medium-rare burger. If you prefer a more well-done burger, grill for another 1 to 2 minutes. Remove the pan from the heat and allow the burgers to rest for 5 minutes.

To build your burger, spread the tzatziki sauce evenly over the bottom half of the buns. Top each bun with a lamb burger, the red onion, arugula and a burger bun top.

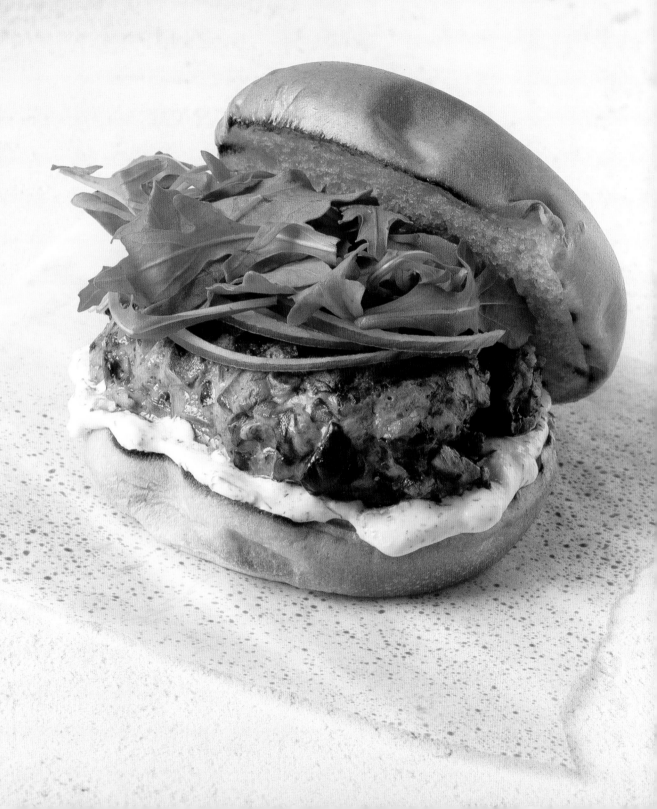

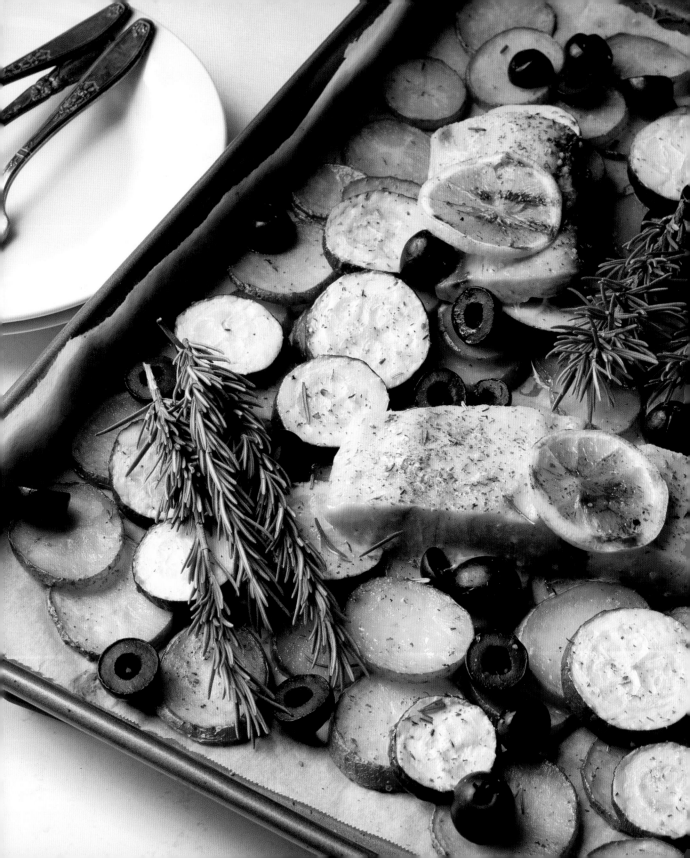

OVEN-ROASTED MAHI-MAHI *with* HERBY POTATOES

MAKES 4 SERVINGS

This dish is a whole meal in one—tender and flaky fish, oven-roasted potatoes and herb-marinated zucchini all cooked on a single pan in the oven. Simply dressed with olive oil, fresh herbs and garlic, it's easy to prepare and perfect for busy weeknight meals. This dish is a great example of how a drizzle of lemon toward the end of cooking can eliminate the need for added salt.

12 oz (340 g) baby red potatoes, cut into round slices

1 large zucchini, cut into round slices

2 tbsp (30 ml) extra virgin olive oil, divided

1 tbsp (2 g) chopped fresh rosemary

2 cloves garlic, minced

4 (3-oz [85-g]) mahi-mahi filets

½ cup (108 g) black pitted olives, cut in half

1 lemon, sliced

Rosemary sprigs, for garnish (optional)

Start by preheating the oven to 350°F (175°C, or gas mark 4). Line a large baking sheet with parchment paper.

In a large bowl, combine the potatoes, zucchini, 1 tablespoon (15 ml) of the olive oil, the rosemary and garlic. Mix well until everything is well coated. Spread the potatoes and zucchini in a single layer on the parchment-lined baking sheet. Place the baking sheet in the oven and roast for 25 minutes, flipping everything over once halfway through the baking time.

Remove the tray from the oven and place the mahi-mahi right on top of the roasted potatoes and zucchini. Scatter the black olives and lemon slices around the pan. Drizzle the remaining olive oil over the fish and roast for 10 minutes in the oven.

Once the fish is cooked through, remove the pan from the oven. Garnish with rosemary sprigs, if desired.

TIP: If you don't have fresh rosemary, you can use dried rosemary in its place. Typically 1 teaspoon of dried herbs is equal to 4 teaspoons (20 g) of fresh herbs.

EASY EGGPLANT STIR-FRY

MAKES 2 SERVINGS

I absolutely love eggplant because it has such a unique flavor and is very filling. This easy stir-fry recipe is another great example of how to apply the principles of the Mediterranean diet: lots of vegetables, a plant-based meal, heart-healthy nuts and plenty of herbs and spices. In this case, I use flavors that aren't traditionally found in the Mediterranean. Cooking the tofu first on its own helps give it some texture so that the shape holds up when added to the stir-fry.

¼ cup (60 ml) low-sodium soy sauce

1 tbsp (15 ml) rice wine vinegar

1 tbsp (15 ml) honey

1 tsp ground ginger

1 tsp cornstarch

3 tbsp (45 ml) extra virgin olive oil, divided

14 oz (396 g) tofu, patted dry with a paper towel and cut into 1-inch (2.5-cm) cubes

1 small eggplant, ends removed and cut into 1-inch (2.5-cm) cubes

4 scallions, green and white parts separated, sliced, divided

2 cloves garlic, minced

½ small jalapeño, diced (seeds removed if you don't like it too spicy)

2 cups (390 g) cooked brown rice

¼ cup (27 g) slivered almonds

In a small bowl, combine the soy sauce, rice wine vinegar, honey and ginger. Stir well to combine, then add in the cornstarch and whisk until incorporated. Set the sauce aside.

In a large cast-iron skillet, heat 1 tablespoon (15 ml) of the olive oil. Add the tofu and cook for 4 minutes on each side. Remove the tofu from the skillet and set it on a plate.

Add the remaining olive oil to the skillet over medium heat. Add the eggplant, white part of the scallions, the garlic and the jalapeño. Cook for 8 to 10 minutes, stirring frequently to prevent the eggplant from sticking to the bottom of the skillet. Add the soy sauce dressing and the tofu to the skillet with the eggplant. Cook for 2 minutes.

Remove the skillet from the heat and serve the stir-fry on top of the brown rice. Garnish with the green parts of the scallions and almonds.

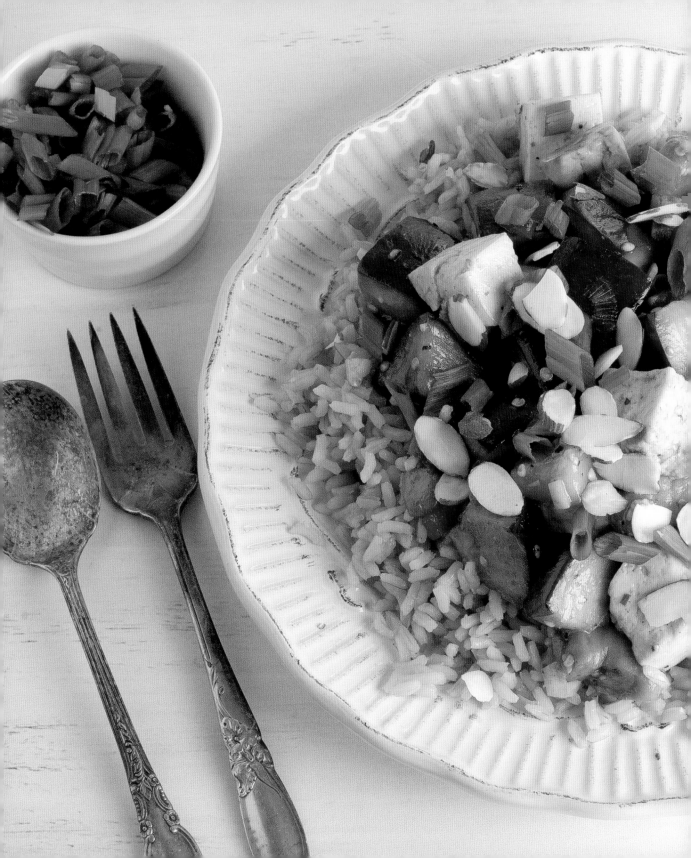

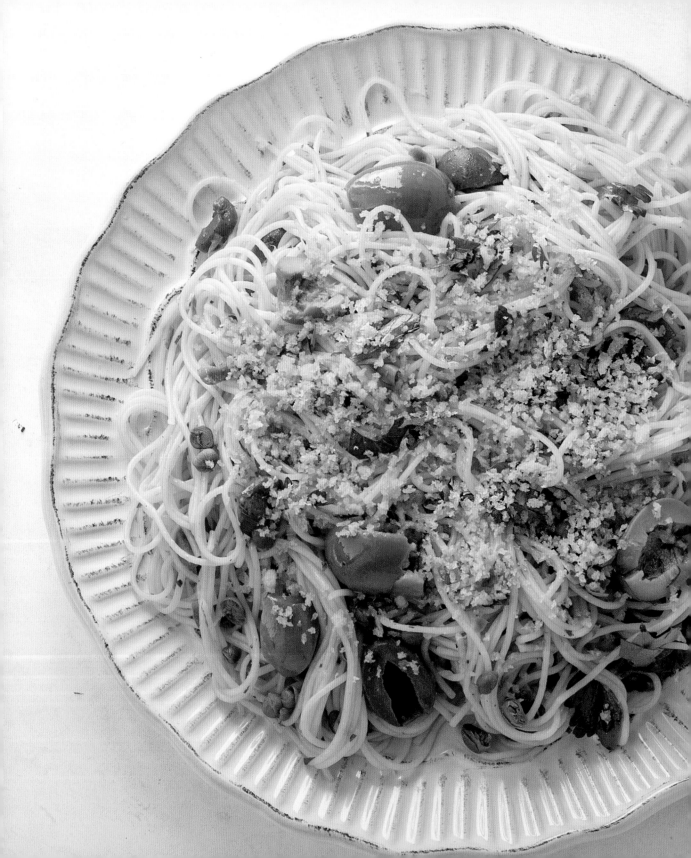

TANGY LINGUINI *with* ANCHOVY *and* TOASTED HERB GREMOLATA

MAKES 4 SERVINGS

I had a dish similar to this recipe in Italy a few years ago and anchovies quickly became one of my favorite ingredients to cook with. They offer the perfect bite of salty, briny flavor and pair so well with the lemon, garlic and herbs. I added some spinach leaves to the anchovy sauce, giving this dish an extra serving of vitamins and minerals.

2 tbsp (30 ml) extra virgin olive oil

½ cup (25 g) panko-style breadcrumbs

1 lemon, zested and juiced, divided

2 cloves garlic, minced, divided

½ cup (30 g) chopped fresh Italian parsley, divided

6 anchovy filets, drained

1 cup (180 g) green olives, pitted and roughly chopped, divided

1 cup (30 g) spinach

2 tbsp (5 g) chopped fresh basil

1 lb (454 g) linguini

¼ cup (25 g) grated Parmesan cheese

In a small skillet, heat the olive oil over medium heat. Once warm, add the breadcrumbs and stir constantly until lightly toasted, about 2 minutes. Remove the skillet from the heat and transfer the toasted breadcrumbs to a small bowl. Add the lemon zest, half of the garlic and ¼ cup (15 g) of parsley. Stir to combine and set it aside.

In a food processor, pulse the anchovy filets until they are finely chopped. Then add the remaining garlic, half of the green olives, the remaining parsley, the spinach and the basil. Pulse all the ingredients together until well combined and finely chopped.

Bring 6 cups (1.5 L) of water to a boil in a large pot. Add the linguini and cook until al dente, about 6 to 7 minutes. Reserve ¼ cup (60 ml) of the water you used to cook the pasta and set it aside before draining the pasta.

Add the drained pasta to a large bowl and add the reserved pasta water and the Parmesan cheese. Stir together and then add the remaining olives, the lemon juice and the anchovy sauce. Mix everything together and top with the herb gremolata.

BRAISED CHICKEN CACCIATORE

Makes 4 servings

There is something so rustic and traditional about this dish that it's one of my favorite recipes to make when we have friends over for dinner. It's hearty and full of wonderful, earthy flavors. I always equate this dish with leisurely dinners spent laughing and talking while simultaneously dipping chunks of crusty bread in the leftover sauce.

1 lb (454 g) chicken thighs, bone-in

½ tsp salt

¼ tsp pepper

1 tbsp (15 ml) extra virgin olive oil

1 medium yellow onion, diced

6 cloves garlic, minced

1 yellow bell pepper, diced

1 red bell pepper, diced

8 oz (227 g) mushrooms, sliced

2 tbsp (38 g) tomato paste

1 (28-oz [794-g]) can crushed tomatoes, drained

2 Roma tomatoes, cut in half

⅔ cup (160 ml) red wine

1 tbsp (5 g) dried oregano

1 tbsp (5 g) dried basil

1 tbsp (3 g) dried thyme

1 (6-oz [170-g]) can black olives, pitted

Lightly season the chicken thighs with the salt and pepper. Then, in a large Dutch oven or ovenproof pot, heat the olive oil over medium heat. Once warm, add the chicken thighs and brown for 5 minutes on each side. Remove them from the skillet and place them on a plate.

In the same skillet, add the onion and sauté until soft and translucent, about 5 to 6 minutes. Add the garlic and sauté while stirring for 30 to 45 seconds.

Add the bell peppers, mushrooms, tomato paste, crushed tomatoes, Roma tomatoes, red wine, oregano, basil and thyme to the pot. Bring these ingredients to a strong simmer, and add the chicken thighs back to the pot. Reduce the heat to low, cover and simmer for 30 minutes, until the chicken is tender and falling off the bone. Add the black olives and simmer for 10 minutes.

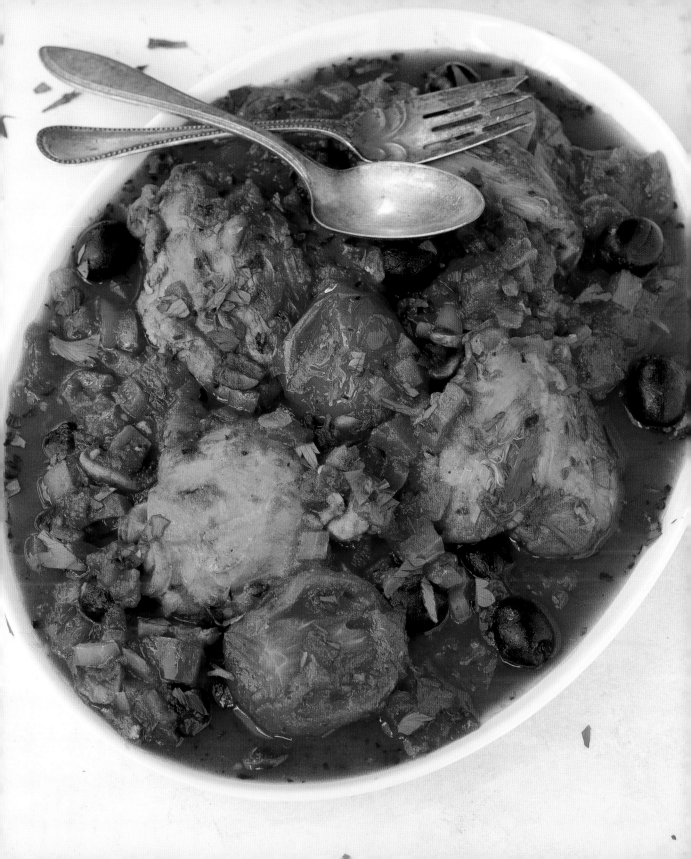

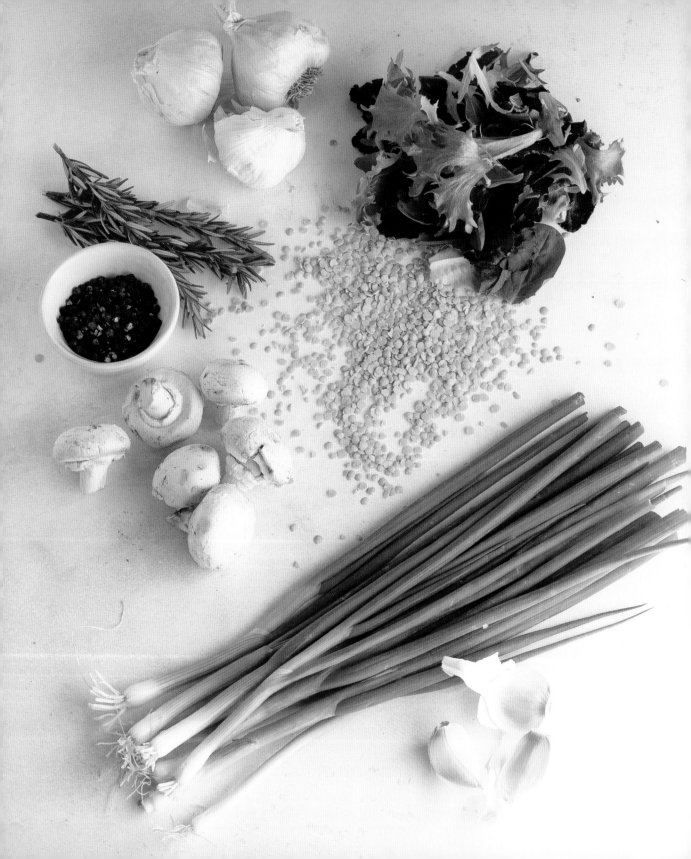

Healthy
SOUPS, SALADS
AND SIDE DISHES

I truly love all the recipes in this book, but this chapter is one of my favorites. I mean who hasn't ordered something off a menu based on the side dishes it comes with?

The key to a good salad, soup or side is that it has to incorporate a lot of flavor and add something to your meal that your main dish may be missing. Maybe that means more vegetables to accompany a more protein-rich dish, or you could pair a smooth and creamy soup with a crispy, crunchy, texture-filled entrée.

The beauty of the recipes in this chapter is that they can accompany an entrée or be enjoyed as a lighter meal. The Hearty Black Bean Soup (page 132) pairs wonderfully with the Simple Herb-Marinated Pork Chops (page 91) or stands alone as a flavorful, hearty, fiber-filled lunch.

This chapter also showcases how simple ingredients can shine when dressed with a little olive oil, such as the Vine-Ripened Tomato and Herb Salad (page 140), or how a humble ingredient like lentils can come alive when tossed in a zesty Dijon dressing (page 127). My time spent in Greece really taught me grains, vegetables, fruits and nuts can be mixed and matched to create amazing dishes that are anything but plain.

The following recipes can also fit into many different seasons based on their ingredients and cooking method. The Refreshing Watermelon Gazpacho Soup (page 144) is the perfect summer no-cook dish, and the Slow Cooker Pasta e Fagioli Soup (page 139) is best on chilly nights in the fall or winter. The Mediterranean diet encourages fresh, locally sourced ingredients whenever possible and this chapter is no exception, especially when it comes to using what's in season throughout the year.

MOROCCAN-SPICED CARROTS

MAKES 4 SERVINGS

I hated carrots growing up–unless they were drowning in ranch dressing. Then I went to Greece and had a roasted carrot dish where the carrots were simply dusted in cinnamon and honey. This is my take on that dish, but with an extra sprinkling of chopped pistachios and fresh herbs. I used colorful petite carrots in this recipe because my daughter thinks they are "cute," but you could easily use regular carrots or even baby carrots.

---

1 lb (454 g) petite carrots, sliced in half

2 tbsp (30 ml) extra virgin olive oil

1 tbsp (15 ml) honey

½ tsp salt

½ tsp pepper

1 tbsp (6 g) orange zest

2 tbsp (30 ml) orange juice

½ tsp cayenne pepper

½ tsp ground cumin

¼ tsp ground cinnamon

¼ cup (4 g) chopped fresh cilantro

1 tbsp (8 g) chopped pistachios

Start by positioning a rack in the center of the oven. Preheat the oven to 400°F (200°C, or gas mark 6). Line a large baking sheet with parchment paper.

In a large mixing bowl, combine the carrots, olive oil, honey, salt and pepper. Mix well with a large spoon or rubber spatula to combine; it will be sticky.

Spread the carrot mixture in a single layer on the parchment-lined baking sheet. Cover the dish lightly with foil and place on the center rack of the oven. Roast for 10 minutes, then remove the foil and roast for 12 to 15 minutes.

While the carrots are roasting, combine the orange zest, orange juice, cayenne pepper, cumin and cinnamon in a small bowl or jar. Set it aside until the carrots are done cooking.

Remove the carrots from the oven and transfer them to a large serving platter. Drizzle them with the orange juice dressing and then garnish with the cilantro and pistachios.

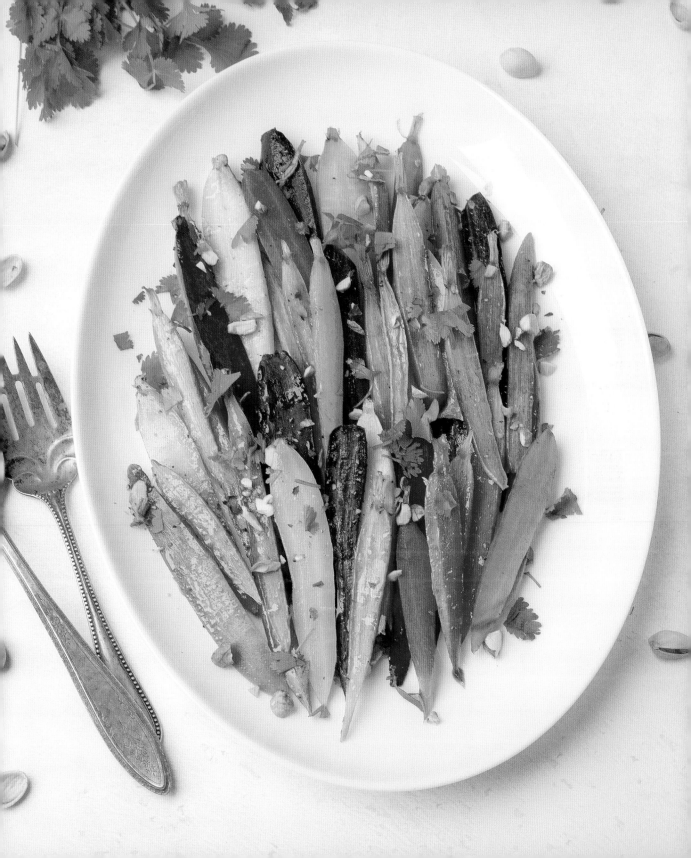

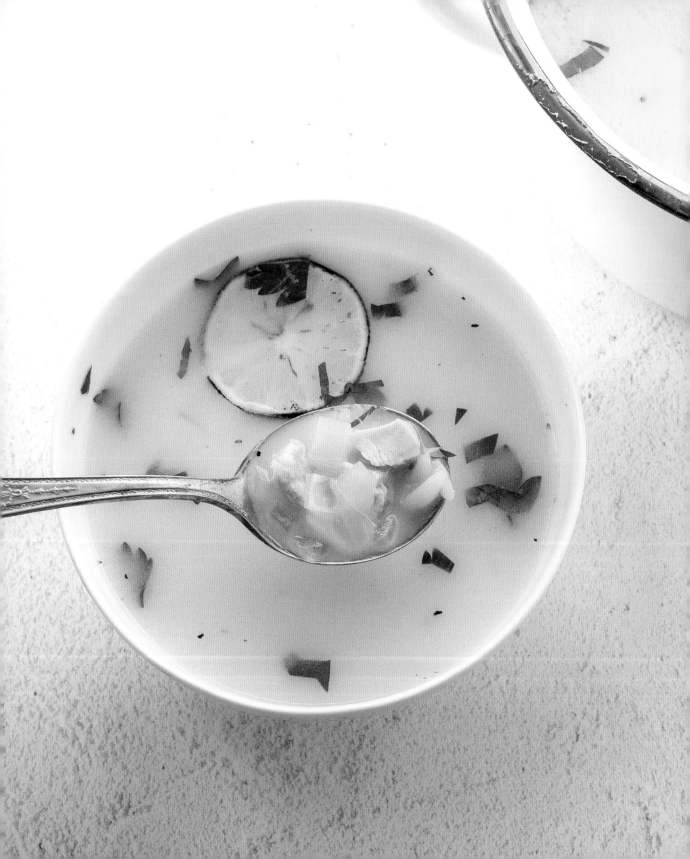

WEEKNIGHT LEMONY CHICKEN ORZO SOUP

Makes 6 servings

This is my go-to dish when I want a warm bowl of soup on a chilly day. It's kind of like a traditional chicken noodle soup but with orzo in place of noodles and an extra burst of flavor from onion, garlic and fresh lemon juice. Stirring the whisked eggs into the hot broth gives the soup an extra thick and creamy texture without needing to add heavy cream.

1 cup (200 g) orzo, uncooked

2 tbsp (30 ml) extra virgin olive oil

½ medium onion, diced

2 cloves garlic, minced

¾ tsp salt

¼ tsp pepper

8 cups (2 L) chicken broth

1 (4-oz [113-g]) chicken breast, cut into 1-inch (2.5-cm) cubes

2 large eggs, at room temperature

⅓ cup (80 ml) fresh lemon juice

¼ cup (15 g) chopped fresh Italian parsley

1 tbsp (15 ml) hot sauce

Sliced lemons, for garnish

In a medium pot, bring 3 cups (720 ml) of water to a boil. Once boiling, add the orzo and cook until tender, about 8 to 9 minutes. Drain and set it aside.

Heat the olive oil in a large soup pot over medium heat. Add the onion and sauté until soft, about 6 minutes. Add the garlic, salt and pepper. Sauté for 3 minutes before adding all 8 cups (2 L) of chicken broth. Bring the broth to a strong boil and then add the chicken. Reduce the heat to a simmer and cook for 20 minutes.

Carefully ladle 1 cup (240 ml) of broth from the soup pot into a small bowl. Whisk in the eggs and lemon juice. Transfer this egg-broth mixture back to the soup pot. Add the cooked orzo, parsley, hot sauce and lemons. Allow the soup to simmer for 2 to 3 minutes before serving.

TIP: This is a great recipe to make if you have leftover roasted chicken on hand. In a pinch, you can use a rotisserie chicken from the store.

GRILLED HALLOUMI *and* FRUIT SALAD *with* HAZELNUTS

MAKES 4 SERVINGS

This fresh and flavor-packed salad is the epitome of balance without skimping on natural, fresh, flavorful ingredients. Juicy, ripe fruit tossed with fresh mint is combined with heart-healthy, crunchy hazelnuts and lightly grilled, slightly salty Halloumi cheese.

Halloumi cheese can be found in the fancy cheese section of most large grocery store chains. The Halloumi itself is a bit salty in flavor, so no additional salt is needed in this recipe.

2 cups (320 g) cantaloupe, either cubed or made into spheres with a melon baller

1 cup (148 g) blueberries

1 tbsp (6 g) chopped fresh mint

2 tbsp (30 ml) extra virgin olive oil

1 tsp pepper

8 oz (227 g) Halloumi, cut into 1-inch (2.5-cm)-thick pieces

2 tbsp (14 g) roughly chopped hazelnuts

In a large bowl, combine the cantaloupe, blueberries, mint, olive oil and pepper. Gently toss to combine and set it aside.

Heat a grill pan or large nonstick pan over medium-high heat. Once hot, add the Halloumi. Allow it to grill without moving or touching it for 5 to 6 minutes on each side. Be sure to cook the Halloumi for at least 5 minutes on each side to ensure that it's cooked correctly. If undercooked, the texture can get a bit rubbery. The outside will be lightly browned from the grill and the inside will be creamy and warm. Carefully remove the Halloumi to a plate and allow it to cool slightly.

On a large serving platter, place your grilled Halloumi and top it with your marinated fruit salad and then garnish with the hazelnuts. Serve immediately.

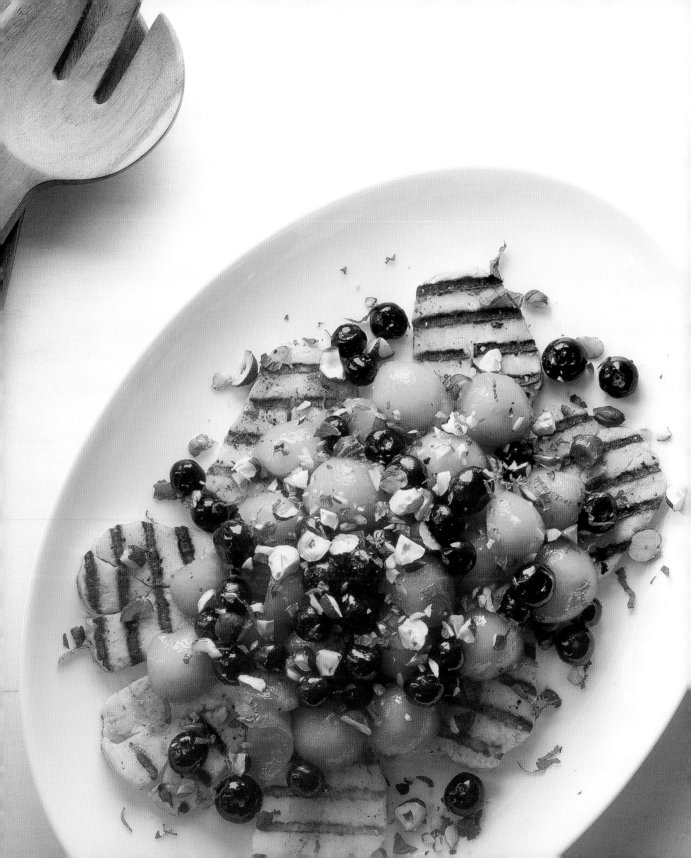

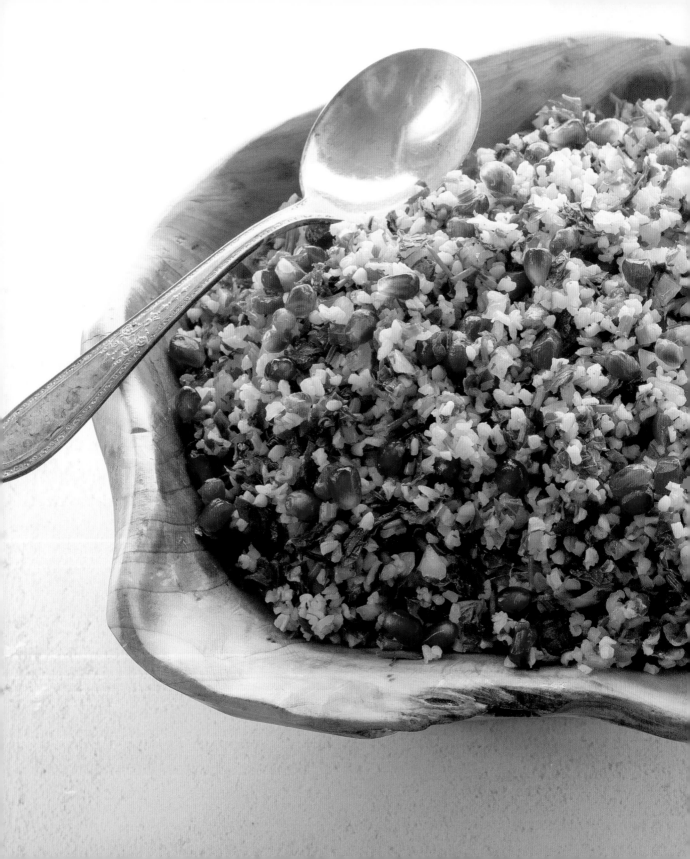

FRESH LEMON *and* HERB TABBOULEH SALAD

MAKES 4 SERVINGS

In my opinion, tabbouleh is one of those foods that pairs well with so many dishes and meals. Besides a bit of chopping, it comes together easily and is made with simple ingredients. The flavors combine for an explosive dish that goes well with chicken, fish, lamb, steak or pork.

Barley is a nutty-flavored grain that brings such a great texture to this dish, in addition to fiber. I like using a food processor to get everything chopped into bite-size pieces, but you could also just use a good old knife and cutting board. This recipe makes great leftovers, so you may want to make extra.

2 cups (480 ml) vegetable broth

1 cup (200 g) barley, uncooked

2 medium Roma tomatoes, roughly chopped

1 cup (60 g) roughly chopped fresh Italian parsley

½ medium onion, peeled and diced

½ cup (46 g) chopped fresh mint

½ cup (120 ml) extra virgin olive oil

3 tbsp (45 ml) fresh lemon juice

1 tsp salt

½ tsp pepper

In a medium pot, bring the vegetable broth and barley to a boil. Once boiling, reduce the heat to low, cover and allow it to simmer for 20 to 30 minutes. You'll want to start checking your barley's texture at about the last 10 minutes of the cooking process. Once most of the liquid has been absorbed, the barley will be doubled in size and become soft and fluffy. Taste to ensure it's completely cooked. Once finished, fluff it with a fork, remove the pot from the heat, cover it again and allow it to sit for 10 minutes to finish absorbing the broth. If there is any liquid left after 10 minutes, you can carefully drain the barley. Set it aside to cool.

Meanwhile, place the tomatoes, parsley, onion and mint in a food processor. Pulse everything together until finely chopped. Add the mixture to a large bowl.

Once cooled, add the cooked barley to the large bowl with the herb mixture. Add the olive oil, lemon juice, salt and pepper, and toss everything together to combine.

TIP: You'll want to cook your barley first so that it has time to cool before putting this recipe together. If you are looking for a timesaving tip, make your barley in advance and keep it in the fridge until you are ready to make this salad.

GOLDEN RICE PILAF

Plain rice is a staple in my home, but it can get a little boring. Luckily, it's easy to switch it up by mixing in different spices or herbs. This simple side dish pairs well with so many recipes, and the turmeric not only gives it a warm spice flavor but a beautiful golden hue as well.

This rice makes a great side dish at dinner and goes great alongside lamb, chicken, steak or pork. This rice also tastes great with dried fruit, such as golden raisins, dried cranberries, currants or apricots. If you are adding dried fruit, toss it directly into the pan with the rice once it's finished cooking, cover and allow to all cook together for an additional 3 minutes.

1½ cups (270 g) basmati rice, uncooked

2 tbsp (30 ml) extra virgin olive oil

1 small onion, finely diced

½ tsp ground cumin

½ tsp ground turmeric

¼ tsp ground cinnamon

2 cloves garlic, minced

¼ tsp salt

¼ tsp pepper

To help ensure that the rice is fluffy rather than mushy once cooked, pour the rice into a fine-mesh strainer and rinse with cold water until the water runs clear.

In a large sauté pan, heat the olive oil over medium heat. Once warm, add the onion and cook until soft, about 4 minutes. Add the cumin, turmeric, cinnamon and garlic to the pan. Stir to combine and sauté for 45 seconds, just until the garlic becomes fragrant.

Add the rinsed basmati rice to the pan and sauté until the rice becomes golden brown, about 3 minutes. Add 2¼ cups (540 ml) of water, the salt and pepper to the pan, and stir to combine. Bring the mixture to a boil, then reduce the heat to low, cover and simmer for 10 to 13 minutes, until all the liquid has been absorbed by the rice.

Remove the pan from the heat and fluff the pilaf lightly with a fork before placing it in a serving bowl.

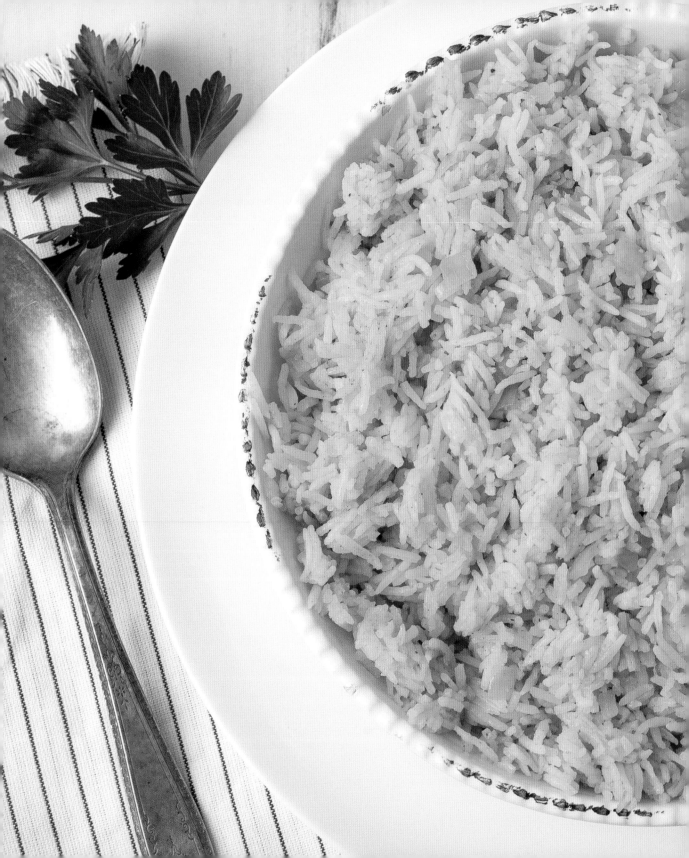

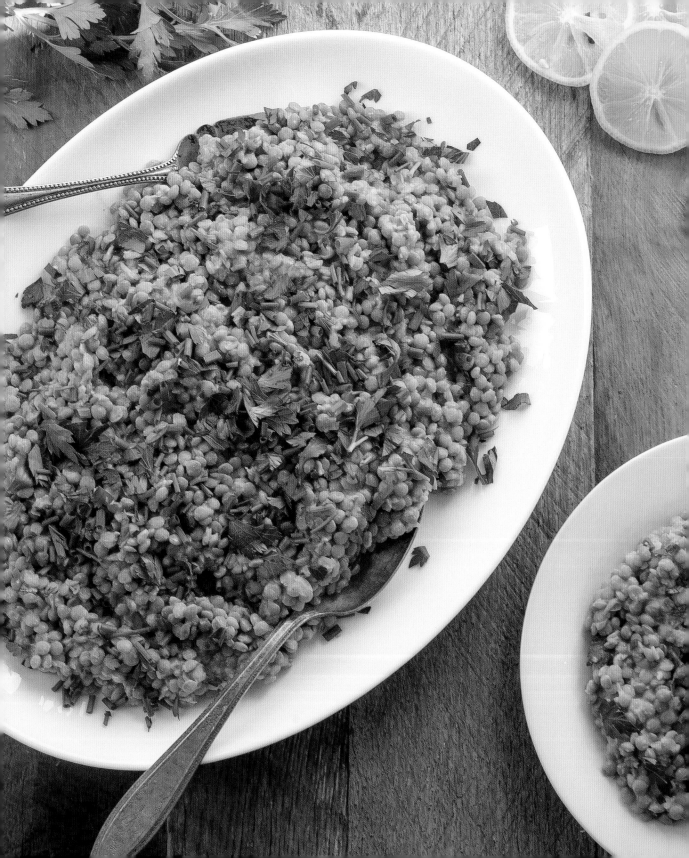

WARM FRENCH LENTIL SALAD *with* DIJON

Lentils are a common ingredient in the Mediterranean diet and for good reason. They are hearty, filling, a good source of plant-based protein and relatively inexpensive. This recipe calls for green lentils because they hold up their shape better when cooked than some other varieties. You could also use pre-cooked lentils found in the produce section of some grocery stores to save yourself even more time. The lentils in this recipe are simply dressed with a warm, zesty, Dijon-based vinaigrette that will have you licking your bowl clean.

2 cups (384 g) small dried green lentils

1 lemon, zested and juiced

4 cloves garlic, minced

3 tbsp (51 g) Dijon mustard

¼ cup (60 ml) extra virgin olive oil

¼ tsp salt

¼ tsp pepper

¼ cup (15 g) chopped fresh Italian parsley

¼ cup (12 g) chopped fresh chives

Place the green lentils in a large pot and cover with 3 cups (720 ml) of water. Bring to a boil, then turn down the heat to low and simmer for about 20 minutes. The lentils should be soft and tender, but not mushy. Once the lentils are cooked, drain them and place them in a large bowl.

While the lentils are cooking, create your Dijon dressing. In a small bowl, combine the lemon zest and juice, garlic, Dijon mustard, olive oil, salt and pepper. Stir well to combine.

Pour the Dijon dressing directly over the bowl of warm, cooked lentils and mix well. Allow the salad to cool just slightly before adding the parsley and chives.

TIP: Buying dried lentils in the bulk bins at most grocery stores is an inexpensive way to purchase only the amount you need.

FARMERS' MARKET PANZANELLA SALAD *with* CREAMY BURRATA

MAKES 4 SERVINGS

This is my favorite recipe to make repeatedly in the late summer, when the tomatoes are huge, juicy and perfectly ripe. It's inspired by the countless panzanella salads I've had while traveling and the beauty of seasonal produce. It features fresh ingredients, olive oil, herbs, lightly toasted bread and a bit of creamy burrata cheese. It's the perfect example of simple ingredients coming together to create a magical dish.

½ crusty baguette, cut into 1-inch (2.5-cm) cubes

2 tbsp (30 ml) extra virgin olive oil

1 tsp Greek Seasoning Spice Blend (page 177)

4 medium heirloom tomatoes, sliced

¼ cup (60 ml) Fresh Herb Oil (page 169), plus more for drizzling

¼ cup (7 g) micro greens or sprouts

1 (2-oz [57-g]) ball fresh burrata cheese

Start by positioning a rack at the top of the oven. Preheat the oven to 375°F (190°C, or gas mark 5). Line a large baking sheet with parchment paper.

In a large bowl, combine the bread, olive oil and Greek seasoning. Combine well so all the bread is coated and then spread it in a thin layer onto the parchment-lined baking sheet. Place the bread on the top rack of the oven and bake for 4 to 5 minutes, until lightly toasted but not as crisp as croutons. Allow the toasted bread to cool slightly.

Place the tomatoes in a large bowl with the cooled, cut bread cubes. Pour the herb oil over the tomatoes and bread. Let the salad sit for about 10 minutes. This will allow the bread to absorb some of the juice from the tomatoes and herb oil, making it even more amazing in every bite.

Finish by topping the tomato salad with the micro greens and place the ball of fresh burrata right in the middle. Drizzle with a little bit of the leftover herb oil, if desired.

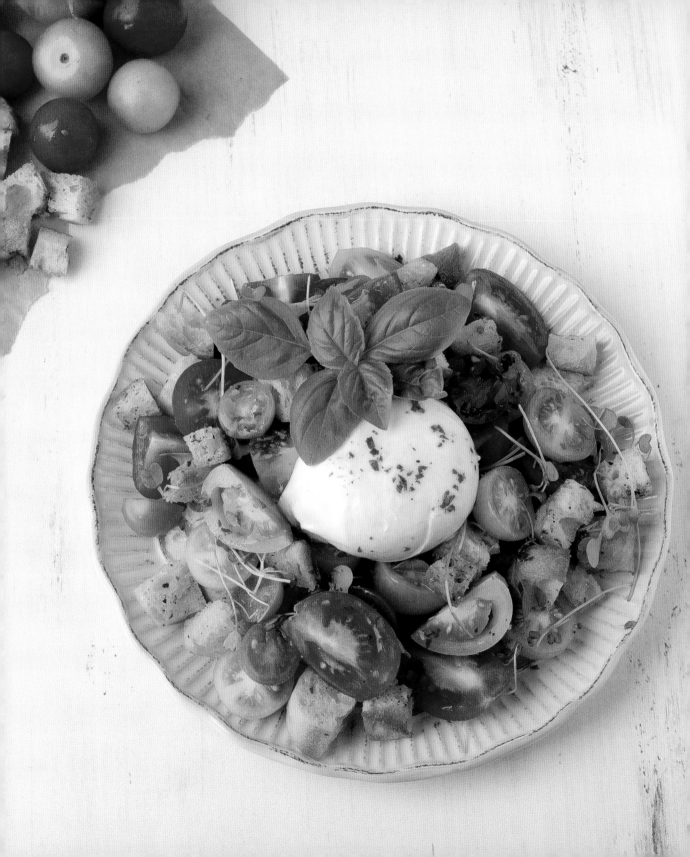

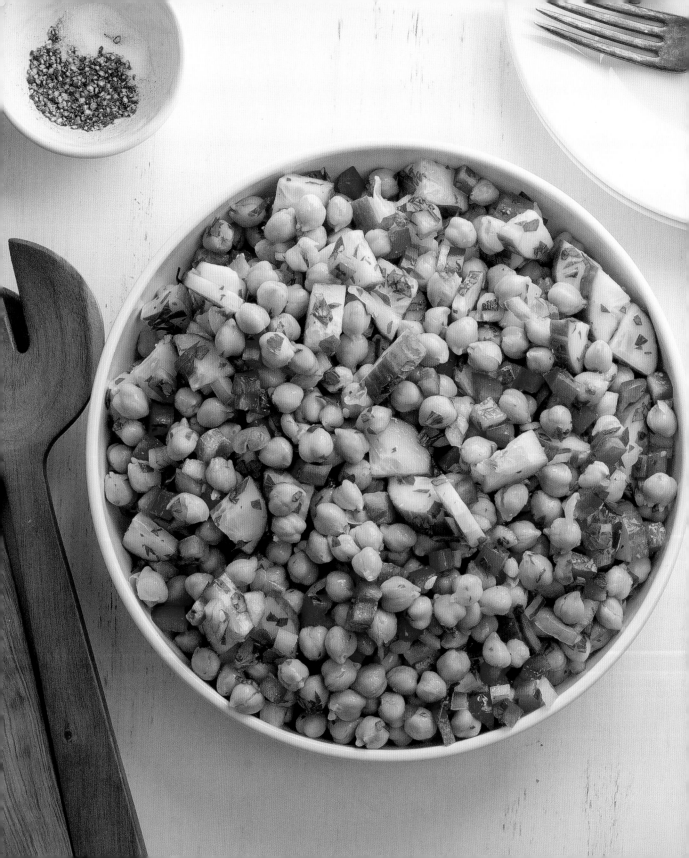

CRUNCHY CHICKPEA SALAD *with* FRESH HERBS

MAKES 4 SERVINGS

This salad is crispy, crunchy and refreshing with a deliciously creamy roasted garlic dressing. It's one of my favorites to prep every Sunday to have in the fridge to serve as a side dish for dinner or as a quick lunch. I love using chickpeas in this salad because they remain crispy on the outside and smooth and creamy on in inside, even when tossed with the dressing. They also are a great plant-based source of protein, as well as a great source of fiber, making them a staple in the Mediterranean diet.

2 (15.5-oz [439-g]) cans chickpeas, drained and rinsed

1 medium cucumber, cut into half-moons

1 red bell pepper, diced

¼ cup (40 g) diced red onion

½ cup (120 ml) Roasted Garlic Dressing (page 178)

1 cup (60 g) chopped fresh Italian parsley

In a large bowl, combine the chickpeas, cucumber, bell pepper and onion. Add the dressing and stir to combine. Top with the parsley. This salad will keep in the fridge for 3 days, making it a great option for meal prep.

TIP: This recipe is fantastic with grilled shrimp or chicken for a more filling meal. If you are pressed for time, you could also use a simple vinaigrette in place of the roasted garlic dressing.

HEARTY BLACK BEAN SOUP

MAKES 8 SERVINGS

Thick, creamy and packed with vegetables, this soup tastes like it's been simmering on the stove for hours, but it actually comes together fairly quickly. It's perfect served alongside roasted chicken or as an accompaniment to a big salad for a lighter lunch or dinner. It also keeps well in the fridge for up to 5 days, making a great leftover lunch.

1 tbsp (15 ml) extra virgin olive oil

1 medium onion, diced

2 ribs celery, diced

2 carrots, peeled and diced

4 cloves garlic, minced

1 bell pepper, diced

4 (15.5-oz [439-g]) cans black beans, drained

4 cups (946 ml) vegetable broth

1 tsp ground cumin

GARNISHES (OPTIONAL)

½ avocado, diced

Juice of 1 lime

¼ cup (38 g) crumbled feta cheese

2 tbsp (6 g) chopped fresh chives

2 tbsp (2 g) chopped fresh cilantro

In a large stockpot, heat the olive oil over medium heat. Add the onion, celery and carrots. Allow the ingredients to sauté until soft, about 10 to 15 minutes. Add the garlic and sauté for 30 to 45 seconds.

Add the bell pepper, black beans, vegetable broth and cumin to the pot. Stir to combine and allow the mixture to come to a boil before reducing the heat to low, covering the pot and allowing the soup to simmer for 20 minutes.

Carefully ladle half of the soup into a blender and puree until smooth. Return the pureed soup back to the pot with the remaining soup and stir to combine. If you have a handheld immersion blender, puree the soup directly in the pot. Be sure to leave it a little on the chunky side instead of completely pureed.

Ladle the soup into serving bowls and top with your desired garnishes—avocado, fresh squeezed lime, feta, chives or cilantro.

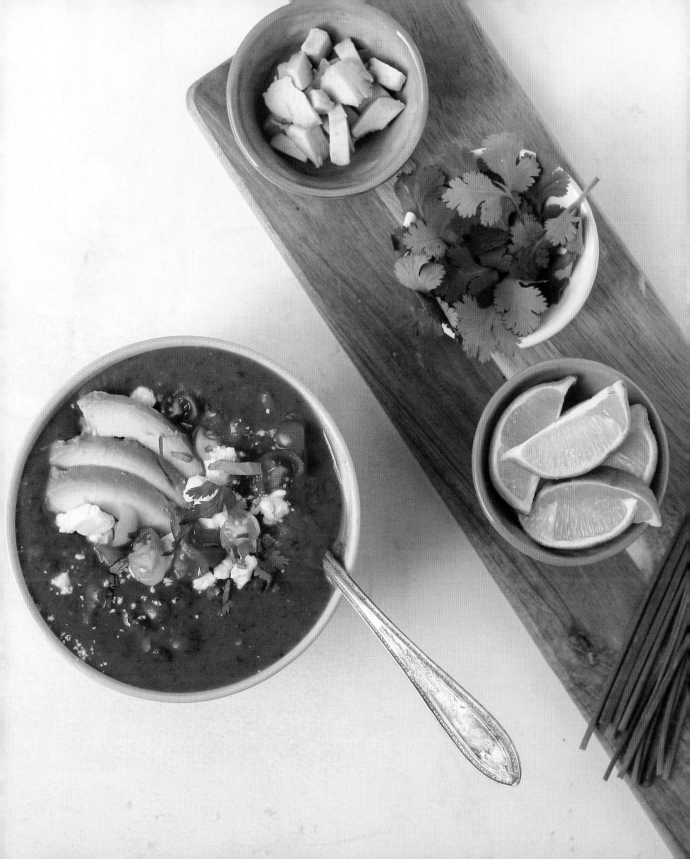

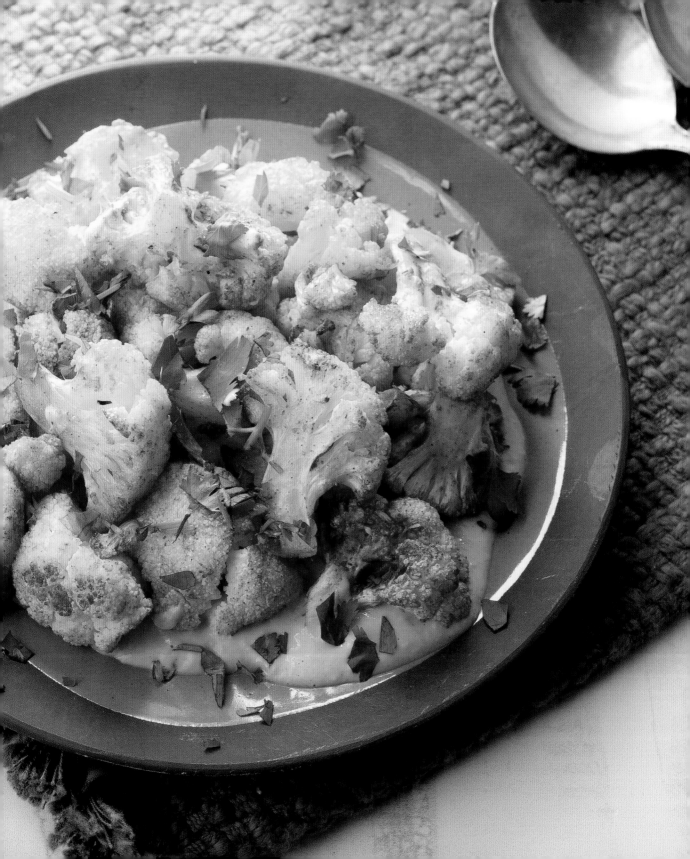

SPICY ROASTED CAULIFLOWER *with* TAHINI DRESSING

MAKES 4 SERVINGS

In this recipe, simple cauliflower combines with a bit of curry and red pepper flakes for a spicy, roasted side dish that is finished off with a tangy tahini sauce and fresh herbs. The key to evenly roasted cauliflower is to preheat the baking sheet in the oven before cooking the cauliflower.

1 head cauliflower, cut into florets

¼ cup (60 ml) extra virgin olive oil

2 tbsp (10 g) curry powder

1 tsp red pepper flakes

½ cup (120 ml) Extra Creamy Tahini Dressing (page 174)

2 tbsp (8 g) chopped fresh Italian parsley

Start by positioning a rack at the top of the oven. Preheat the oven to 425°F (220°C, or gas mark 6). Once the oven is warm, preheat a large baking sheet in the oven for 5 to 10 minutes. This will help ensure the cauliflower gets nice and roasted on all sides.

In a large bowl, combine the cauliflower florets, olive oil, curry powder and red pepper flakes. Mix until all of the cauliflower is well coated.

Transfer the cauliflower mixture to your preheated baking sheet and spread it out in an even, single layer. Place the sheet on the top rack of the oven and roast for 20 to 25 minutes. Flip the cauliflower over halfway through the cooking process.

Once the cauliflower is finished roasting, it will be a beautiful golden color with slightly charred edges. Remove the baking sheet from the oven and allow the cauliflower to cool slightly.

Place the dressing on the bottom of a serving dish. Top with the roasted cauliflower and garnish with parsley.

TIP: If you are pressed for time, you can buy precut cauliflower florets.

SHAVED BRUSSELS SPROUT SALAD *with* PARMESAN

MAKES 6 SERVINGS

This is so light and simple: Thinly shaved Brussels sprouts are tossed with a creamy garlic dressing. Then the salad is combined with crunchy hazelnuts and almonds and a sprinkling of Parmesan cheese for a filling and flavorful dish. I love recipes like this that really show how simple ingredients can come together to create dishes that are big on flavor but easy to create at home.

1 lb (454 g) Brussels sprouts

⅓ cup (38 g) roughly chopped hazelnuts

⅓ cup (48 g) roughly chopped almonds

⅓ cup (80 ml) Roasted Garlic Dressing (page 178)

¼ cup (25 g) freshly grated Parmesan cheese

Using a box grater, carefully shave the Brussels sprouts. You could also cut off the bottoms and place them in a food processor to chop. You just want to ensure the Brussels sprouts are thinly chopped.

Place the shaved Brussels sprouts in a large bowl and add the hazelnuts, almonds and dressing. Mix well to combine. Top the salad with the Parmesan cheese.

TIP: Some stores sell thinly shaved Brussels sprouts in the produce section. They work wonderfully in this recipe.

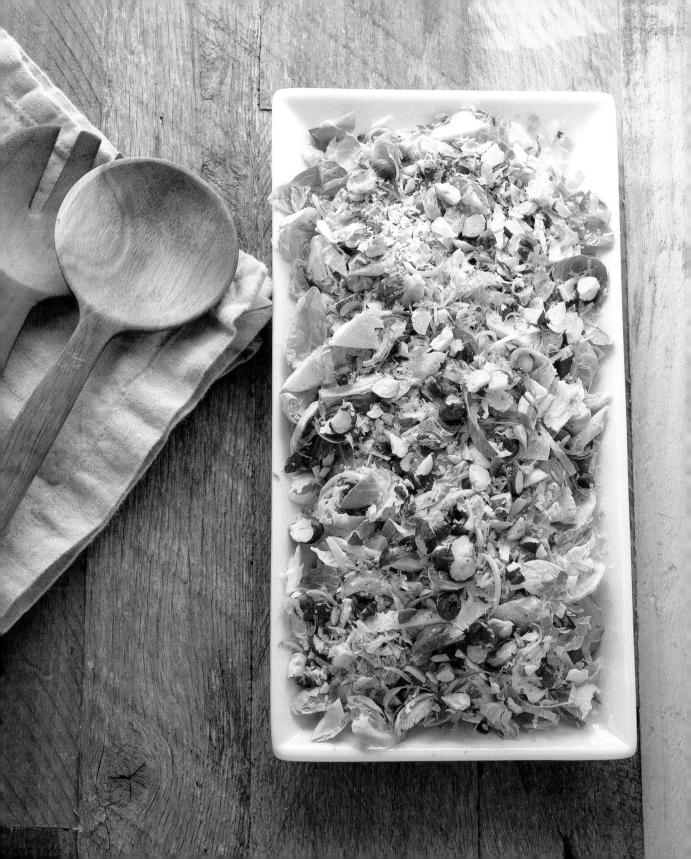

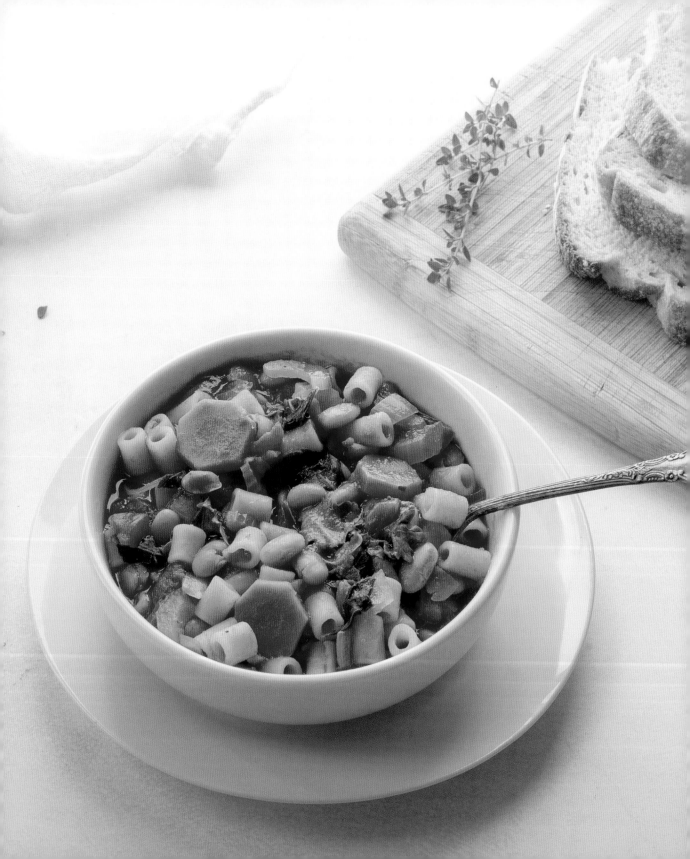

SLOW COOKER PASTA E FAGIOLI SOUP

MAKES 6 SERVINGS

There is nothing easier than throwing a handful of ingredients in a slow cooker, setting the timer and coming home to a warm, hearty bowl of soup. This recipe features fresh vegetables, canned beans, garlic, a touch of white wine and the secret weapon to flavorful, creamy soup—the rind of fresh Parmesan cheese. It slowly melts into the soup as it cooks, infusing so much flavor. If you can't find the rind, you can easily substitute in Parmesan cheese.

1 (28-oz [794-g]) can crushed tomatoes with liquid

1 medium yellow onion, diced

1 (15.5-oz [439-g]) can cannellini beans, drained and rinsed

3 carrots, peeled and diced

3 ribs celery, diced

4 cloves garlic, minced

1 small Parmesan cheese rind (can substitute ½ cup [50 g] of Parmesan cheese)

½ cup (120 ml) dry white wine

4 cups (946 ml) vegetable broth

2 cups (210 g) macaroni pasta

2 cups (134 g) roughly chopped kale

In the inner pot of your slow cooker, combine the crushed tomatoes, onion, beans, carrots, celery, garlic, Parmesan cheese rind, white wine and vegetable broth. Set the slow cooker to low and cook for 8 hours.

After 8 hours, add the pasta and kale to the slow cooker. Cover and cook for 30 minutes, until the pasta is cooked through.

VINE-RIPENED TOMATO *and* HERB SALAD

MAKES 4 SERVINGS

The epitome of summer in a bowl: This dish is easy, fresh and packed with basil, parsley and mint. The salad is simply dressed with olive oil, honey, lemon and shallot, and that allows all the natural flavors of the ingredients to shine through. Perfect for backyard dinner parties in the summer or a quick side dish to accompany grilled fish or chicken.

2 lb (907 g) vine-ripened tomatoes, quartered

¼ cup (10 g) chopped fresh basil

¼ cup (15 g) chopped fresh Italian parsley

2 tbsp (11 g) chopped fresh mint

2 tbsp (17 g) sunflower seeds

1 small shallot, diced

⅓ cup (80 ml) extra virgin olive oil

⅛ cup (30 ml) red wine vinegar

1 tsp fresh lemon juice

½ tsp honey

In a large bowl, combine the tomatoes, basil, parsley, mint and sunflower seeds. Set it aside.

In a small bowl or jar, combine the shallot, olive oil, red wine vinegar, lemon juice and honey. Whisk together until the dressing is well combined.

Pour the dressing over the salad. Mix until well combined. This salad is best if you allow it to sit and marinate for 30 minutes before serving.

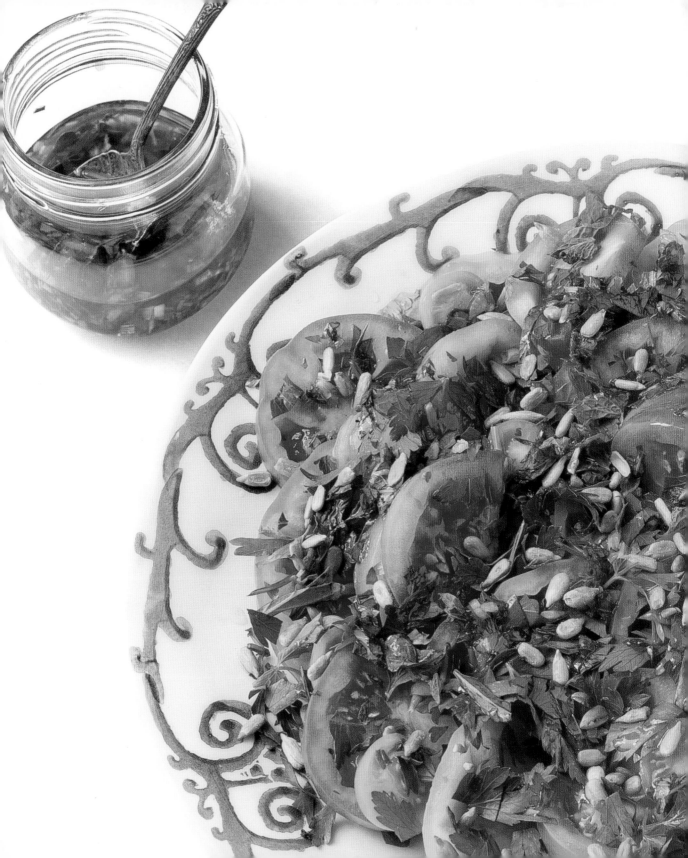

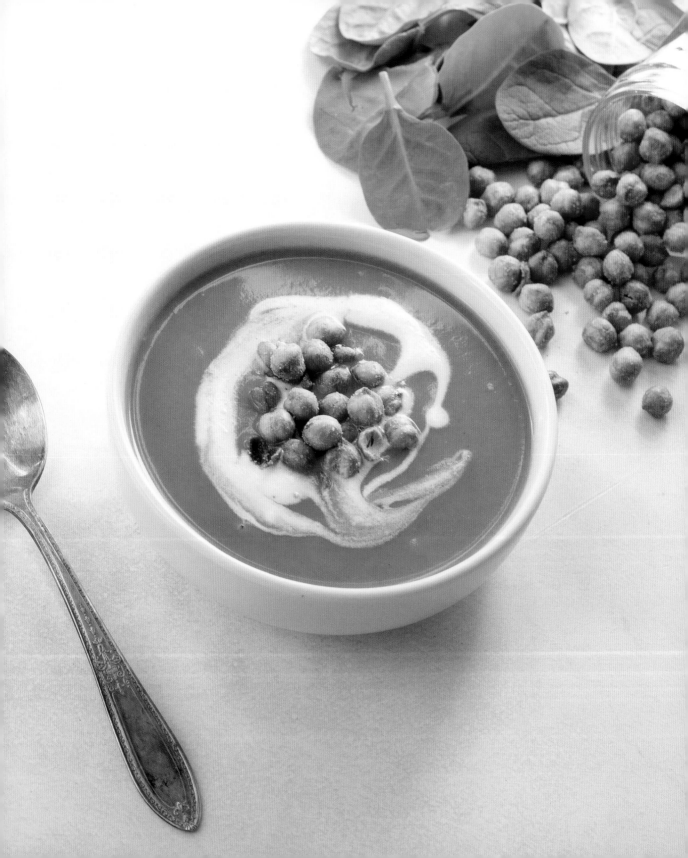

CREAMY SPINACH *and* CAULIFLOWER SOUP *with* SPICED CHICKPEAS

MAKES 6 SERVINGS

Vibrant spinach and hearty cauliflower combine to create a deliciously creamy soup that is finished off with a touch of Greek yogurt, fresh lemon juice and crispy spiced chickpeas. It's warm, filling and tastes so rich that you won't believe it doesn't contain cream. The crispy chickpeas make a great snack if you have extra.

1 (15.5-oz [439-g]) can chickpeas, drained and rinsed

3 tbsp (45 ml) extra virgin olive oil, divided

½ tsp salt

1 tsp paprika

1 tsp ground turmeric

1 medium onion, chopped

3 cloves garlic, roughly chopped

3 scallions, green and white parts, sliced

¼ cup (13 g) chopped fresh dill

1 head cauliflower, cut into florets

4 cups (946 ml) vegetable broth

6 oz (170 g) spinach

2 tbsp (30 ml) fresh lemon juice

½ cup (120 ml) plain Greek yogurt

Start by preheating the oven to 350°F (175°C, or gas mark 4).

After draining and rinsing the chickpeas, pat them dry with a paper towel. Roll the beans between two towels and remove the skins that break loose. The more skins that you remove, the crispier your chickpeas will be once cooked.

Place the chickpeas in a small bowl and add 1 tablespoon (15 ml) of the olive oil and the salt. Spread the chickpeas in a single layer on a large baking sheet and place it in the oven to bake for 45 to 60 minutes. Shake the sheet halfway through the baking time. When the chickpeas are done cooking, remove the baking sheet from the oven and sprinkle the chickpeas with the paprika and ground turmeric. Allow them to cool.

In a large pot over medium heat, heat 1 tablespoon (15 ml) of olive oil. Add the onion and sauté for 5 minutes, stirring frequently. Add the garlic, scallions and dill to the pot. Sauté for 2 minutes before adding the cauliflower florets and vegetable broth. Bring the mixture to a boil, then cover and reduce to a simmer for 25 minutes.

Once the soup has simmered, add the spinach and stir until the spinach is wilted, about 3 minutes. Use a ladle to transfer the soup to a blender. Add the lemon juice and Greek yogurt to the blender, and puree until the soup is smooth and creamy. Serve in bowls with the remaining olive oil drizzled over the soup and topped with some crispy chickpeas.

REFRESHING WATERMELON GAZPACHO SOUP

MAKES 4 SERVINGS

This chilled soup is creamy, smooth and slightly sweet with the perfect bit of kick to wake up your taste buds. It's amazing in the summer when watermelon and tomatoes are at their seasonal peak. Using seasonal produce is a great way to ensure you get the best flavor and ripest produce, often at the best price.

This chilled soup is perfect to enjoy on a warm evening at the start of a dinner and is great to make when sharing a meal with loved ones because it can be easily made in a big batch.

2 cups (304 g) watermelon, cut into chunks

2 medium tomatoes, quartered

1 medium cucumber, peeled and chopped

½ small jalapeño, seeds removed and diced

3 tbsp (45 ml) extra virgin olive oil, divided

1 tsp sherry vinegar

¼ tsp salt

¼ tsp pepper

½ cup (18 g or about one slice) chopped sourdough bread, crust removed

Fresh basil, diced cucumber and diced tomato, for garnish (optional)

In a large blender, place the watermelon, tomatoes, cucumber and jalapeño. Blend until well pureed and smooth in texture. Add 2 tablespoons (30 ml) of the olive oil, the sherry vinegar, salt and pepper. Puree again until well combined.

Transfer the mixture to a large bowl and add the sourdough bread. Cover the bowl and place it in the fridge for 4 hours, then transfer the mixture back to the blender and puree once more until thick and creamy.

Ladle into serving bowls and drizzle with the remaining olive oil. Garnish with basil, cucumber and tomato, if desired.

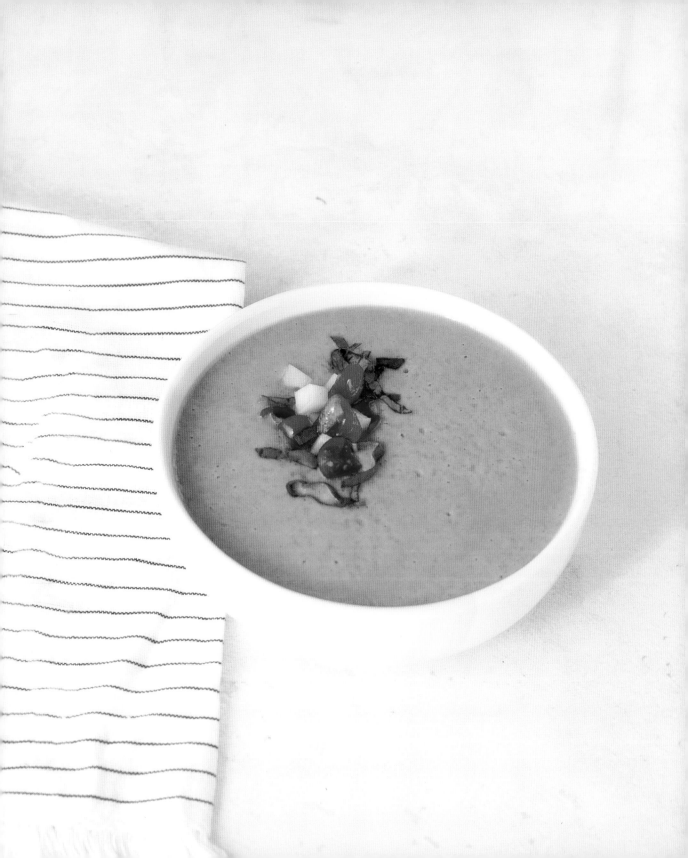

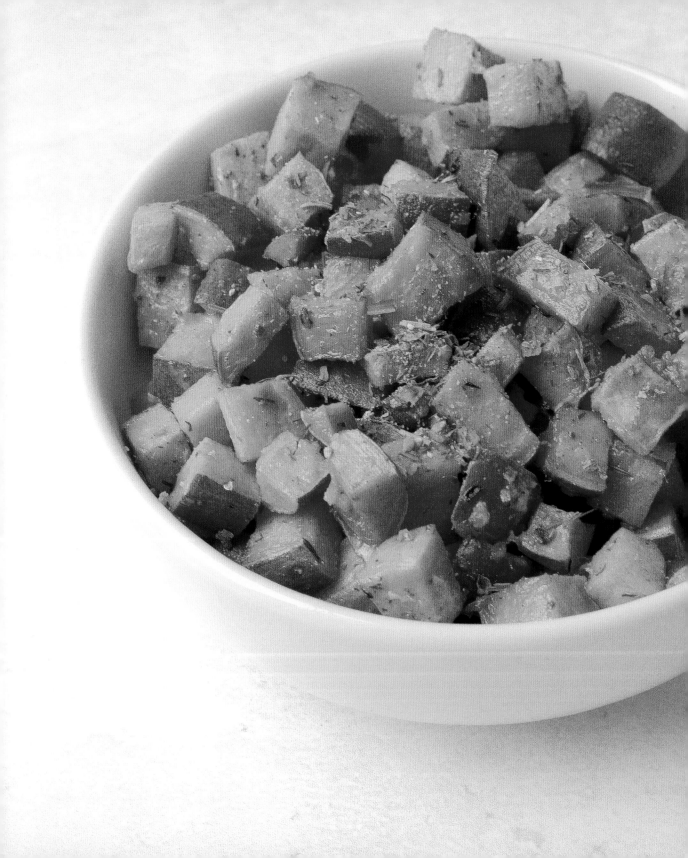

PARMESAN *and* GARLIC ROASTED SWEET POTATOES

MAKES 3 SERVINGS

Sweet potatoes are packed full of nutrients and are a hearty ingredient that can be added to many meals. Roasting them in the oven creates a crispy outside with a warm and creamy interior. Flavored here with just a bit of olive oil, garlic, Greek seasoning and Parmesan cheese, they are the perfect side to any entrée. I love making a double batch of these roasted sweet potatoes and enjoying them the following day for breakfast, warmed and topped with a fried egg.

3 cups (400 g) diced sweet potatoes

2 tbsp (30 ml) extra virgin olive oil

3 cloves garlic, minced

¼ cup (25 g) grated Parmesan cheese

1 tsp Greek Seasoning Spice Blend (page 177)

Start by positioning a rack in the center of the oven. Preheat the oven to 400°F (200°C, or gas mark 6). Line a large baking sheet with parchment paper.

In a large bowl, combine the sweet potatoes, olive oil, garlic, Parmesan cheese and Greek seasoning. Mix well to combine.

Spread the sweet potato mixture in a single layer on the parchment-lined baking sheet. Place the baking sheet on the center rack of the oven and bake for 20 to 25 minutes. The potatoes will be lightly caramelized on the outside and tender on the inside when fully cooked. You should be able to easily pierce them with a fork when done.

Remove the baking sheet from the oven and allow the sweet potatoes to cool slightly before serving.

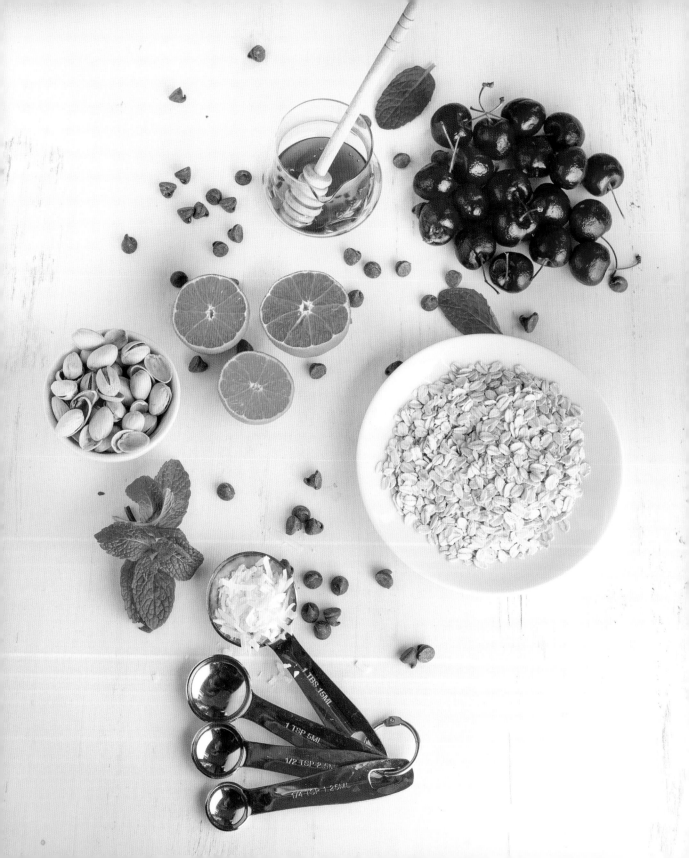

Simple
SWEETS
AND TREATS

I have always had a major sweet tooth and that hasn't faded as I've grown. Part of my love of the Mediterranean diet is that there isn't anything that is off limits, including desserts. It's more about balance, portion size and using real ingredients to create sweets and treats.

The key is to incorporate desserts into your lifestyle that aren't created with tons of extra sugar, heavy cream or butter. An easy way to do this is to rely on the sweetness of real fruit and use the heartiness and creamy texture of nuts and olive oil in place of butter if possible. You'll be surprised how much flavor and satisfaction you can get when treats are prepared simply and in the right flavor combinations—without any need for an excess of added sugars, butter or artificial ingredients.

If you are looking for something chocolatey, the Peanut Butter and Chocolate Walnut Bites (page 154) are the perfect choice. They'll satisfy your craving for rich and decadent-tasting chocolate, with the benefits of real ingredients such as cocoa powder, coconut and honey. If sweet desserts are more your thing, the Grilled Strawberries with Mint and Yogurt (page 153) are naturally sweet and creamy at the same time. They're refreshing and will satisfy even the biggest sweet tooth.

Of course the occasional indulgence of a heavenly slice of chocolate cake or freshly baked cookie should be enjoyed and never be a cause of guilt. One of my favorite tips is to split a rich dessert with friends at the end of the meal.

3-INGREDIENT CANTALOUPE SORBET

MAKES 8 SERVINGS

Sorbet is such a refreshing dessert, especially on warm summer nights. I prepare it with ripe, fresh fruit that I freeze in chunks; this creates a creamier sorbet. Cantaloupe is delicious, or you can easily substitute your favorite summer fruit. Try strawberries, raspberries or peaches. This is perfect to enjoy after a delicious meal, when you just want a hint of something sweet without it being too heavy or rich.

1 medium cantaloupe, cubed

1 tbsp (15 ml) fresh lemon juice

1 tbsp (15 ml) honey

Line a large baking sheet with parchment paper. Place the cantaloupe in a single layer on the lined baking sheet and place it in the freezer for 2 to 3 hours.

Once frozen, place the cantaloupe cubes in a blender with the lemon juice and honey. Puree until thick and creamy. If you noticed your sorbet is too thick, add a little bit of water to help the mixture puree smoothly.

Place the pureed sorbet in a freezer-friendly dish and store it in the freezer if not serving immediately. Before serving, you will need to let the sorbet sit at room temperature for about 3 to 5 minutes to soften.

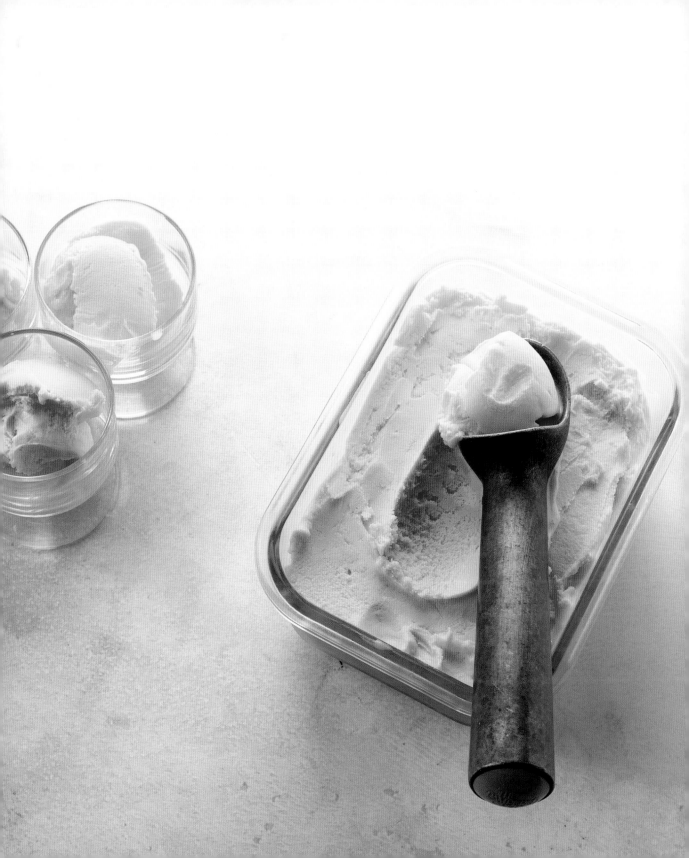

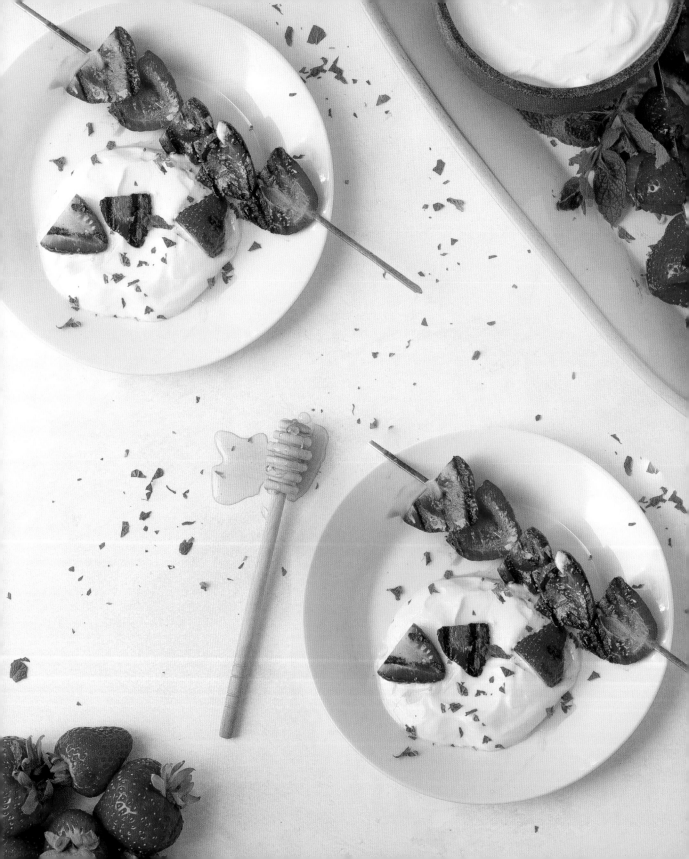

GRILLED STRAWBERRIES *with* MINT *and* YOGURT

MAKES 2 SERVINGS

Grilling fruit is an easy way to bring out natural sweetness and elevate an otherwise ordinary dish. This recipe features fresh strawberries, served on top of creamy Greek yogurt, with a drizzle of honey and a little mint. If you don't like strawberries or they aren't in season, pineapple, peaches or plums would work well in this recipe. In Greece, dessert is commonly some sort of fruit served with either a single scoop of ice cream or creamy yogurt. It is simple but so fresh and light.

16 large strawberries, hulled and cut in half

½ cup (120 ml) plain Greek yogurt

1 tbsp (15 ml) honey

1 tbsp (6 g) chopped fresh mint

Preheat a grill pan over medium-high heat. While it's warming up, thread 8 strawberry halves onto four wooden or metal skewers.

Once the grill is warm, place each skewer gently on top and grill for 2 to 3 minutes on each side. Be very careful when turning over the skewers as they may be warm. Remove the pan from the heat and allow the berries to cool slightly.

Divide the Greek yogurt evenly onto two serving plates. Then place two grilled strawberry skewers on each plate, drizzle with the honey and garnish with the fresh mint.

TIP: If you are using wooden skewers, soak them in water for about 5 to 10 minutes before using. This will help prevent any wood from splintering off or burning.

PEANUT BUTTER *and* CHOCOLATE WALNUT BITES

MAKES 12 BITES

Is there any flavor combo out there as good as peanut butter and chocolate? These decadent-tasting sweets are the perfect bite of creamy peanut butter, rich cocoa, crunchy walnuts and a touch of honey. Even better, they can be made in advance and stored in the freezer for a quick pop of chocolate when the craving hits.

½ cup (130 g) peanut butter

3 tbsp (45 ml) honey

1 tsp vanilla extract

3 tbsp (21 g) unsweetened cocoa powder

½ cup (59 g) walnuts

½ cup (47 g) unsweetened coconut flakes

Powdered sugar, for garnish (optional)

In a mixing bowl, combine the peanut butter, honey, vanilla and cocoa powder. Use an electric mixer to mix until everything is well combined and creamy, about 2 minutes. If the mixture is too thick, add 1 tablespoon (15 ml) of warm water to loosen. The mixture will resemble the consistency of thick frosting.

In a food processor, pulse the walnuts until they form a fine flour-like consistency. Add this walnut mixture to the mixing bowl. Mix on low speed until well combined. Stir in the coconut. Set the bowl in the fridge for 20 minutes, just until the mixture is set and easier to work with.

Using a small scoop, form 12 balls by rolling the mixture with your hands into a compact bite-size ball and place them on a serving plate. Garnish with powdered sugar, if desired.

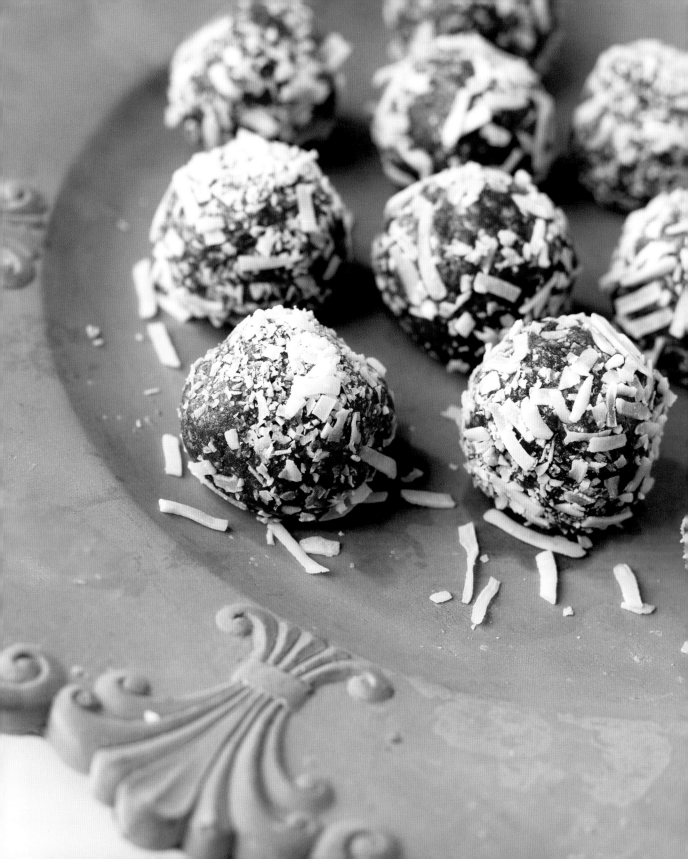

ALMOND *and* CHERRY BAKED BISCOTTI

MAKES 18 TO 20 BISCOTTI

There is something so delicious about homemade biscotti dipped into a freshly brewed cup of coffee, and now you can indulge in that small little treat in your own home. Making biscotti may seem daunting at first, but the recipe is very forgiving and so worth the little bit of extra time it takes to prepare.

1⅓ cups (191 g) almonds, divided

1¾ cups (219 g) all-purpose flour

2 tsp (9 g) baking powder

¼ tsp salt

2 large eggs

1 cup (200 g) sugar

4 tbsp (56 g) butter, melted

1 tsp almond extract

1 cup (131 g) dried cherries

Olive oil cooking spray

1 egg white, lightly whisked in a small bowl

Start by positioning a rack in the center of the oven. Preheat the oven to 350°F (175°C, or gas mark 4). Line a large baking sheet with parchment paper.

In a large food processor, pulse 1 cup (143 g) of the almonds until they are coarsely chopped; this is about six pulses on the food processor. Transfer the chopped almonds to a bowl and set it aside.

In the empty food processor, add the remaining ⅓ cup (48 g) of almonds and process them until they are finely ground. Add the flour, baking powder and salt. Mix the ingredients together in the food processor until combined, about 30 seconds. Transfer this mixture to the bowl with the coarsely chopped almonds. Stir to combine.

Crack the eggs into the food processor and puree at a constant speed until the eggs become very light in color and double in size; this will take about 3 to 4 minutes. Working very slowly, add the sugar to the eggs while the food processor is still running. Add the melted butter and almond extract to the food processor. Mix everything together until well combined, about 20 seconds. Transfer the egg mixture to a large mixing bowl.

Slowly add half of the flour-almond mixture to the mixing bowl with the eggs and gently fold together using a rubber spatula until they are just combined; be careful not overmix during this step. Add the remaining flour-almond mixture to the bowl, along with the dried cherries. Fold everything together gently until combined and a dough forms.

To form the two loaves that will become your biscotti, lightly flour your hands to ensure the dough doesn't stick to your fingers. Gently divide the dough in half with your hands. Form each half into a rectangle that is roughly 7 x 3 inches (18 x 7.5 cm) in size on the parchment-lined baking sheet. Spray the top of each loaf with olive oil cooking spray and use a rubber spatula to lightly smooth the surface. Gently brush the top of each loaf with the egg white.

Place the baking sheet in the oven and bake for 20 to 25 minutes, until the loaves are golden brown and starting to gently crack on the surface. Remove the baking sheet from the oven and allow the loaves to cool for 30 minutes.

Place the cooled loaves on a large cutting board and use a serrated knife to cut each loaf into ½-inch (1-cm)-thick pieces, being sure to cut on the bias to form long biscotti slices. Place a wire rack over the parchment-lined baking sheet and carefully arrange the biscotti slices in a single layer on the wire rack.

Place the biscotti back in the oven, reduce the oven temperature to 325°F (170°C, or gas mark 3) and bake for 30 minutes, flipping the biscotti over halfway through the baking time. Once done, the biscotti will be dark brown in color. Allow the biscotti to cool completely before serving.

*See photo on page 2.

TIP: These biscotti make wonderful gifts during the holidays.

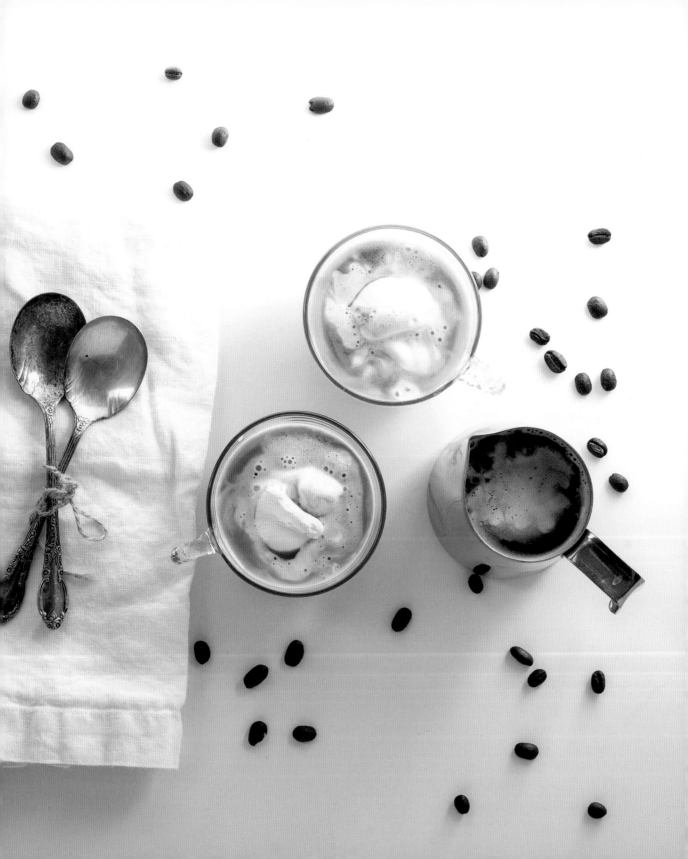

TRADITIONAL AFFOGATO *with* CREAMY VANILLA ICE CREAM

MAKES 2 SERVINGS

The first time I ever had an affogato, I had just finished an absolutely wonderful meal in Italy. I wasn't really hungry for anything sweet, so the waiter suggested an affogato to finish off the meal. Coffee is a respected tradition throughout the Mediterranean and differs slightly from region to region. It's rarely taken "to go" and instead meant to be sipped and enjoyed, typically with friends or family.

I was skeptical at first about pouring hot espresso over ice cream, but it has since become one of my favorite after-dinner treats. You can also switch up the ice cream flavor. One of my favorites is salted caramel ice cream.

2 scoops vanilla ice cream

4 tbsp (60 ml) freshly brewed espresso

Place the scoop of vanilla ice cream in a small bowl or glass. Slowly pour the freshly brewed espresso over the ice cream. Serve immediately.

TIP: Making espresso at home requires some type of espresso machine or other equipment. There are many options available from traditional Italian-style espresso machines, smaller countertop versions and trendy pod-style espresso makers, to stovetop methods like a Moka pot.

LIGHT *and* LEMONY OLIVE OIL CAKE

MAKES 8 TO 10 SLICES

This recipe was inspired by my grandma (Hi, Oma). She never failed to have a coffee cake on hand when people stopped by to visit. This cake is made with olive oil in place of butter and unsweetened applesauce replaces half of the sugar. The end result is a light, buttery cake with just a hint of lemon that's perfect with a cup of coffee or tea.

3 large eggs

¼ cup (50 g) sugar

½ cup (128 g) unsweetened applesauce

¼ cup (60 ml) plus 1 tbsp (15 ml) extra virgin olive oil, divided

½ cup (120 ml) milk

1 tbsp (15 ml) fresh lemon juice

1 tsp vanilla extract

1½ cups (188 g) all-purpose flour

1½ tsp (7 g) baking powder

½ tsp salt

Start by positioning a rack in the center of the oven. Preheat the oven to 350°F (175°C, or gas mark 4). Spray an 8-inch (20-cm) round cake pan with nonstick cooking spray. Line the bottom of the pan with parchment paper.

In a large bowl, use an electric mixer to beat together the eggs and sugar for 30 seconds. Add the applesauce and mix for 30 seconds.

Beat in the ¼ cup (60 ml) of olive oil in a slow, steady stream on medium speed. Add the milk, lemon juice and vanilla, and mix together until just combined.

In a separate bowl, sift together the flour, baking powder and salt. Gradually add the flour mixture to the egg mixture. Stir gently to combine.

Pour the batter into the prepared cake pan and bake on the center rack of the oven for 30 minutes.

Brush the top of the cake with the remaining olive oil just before serving.

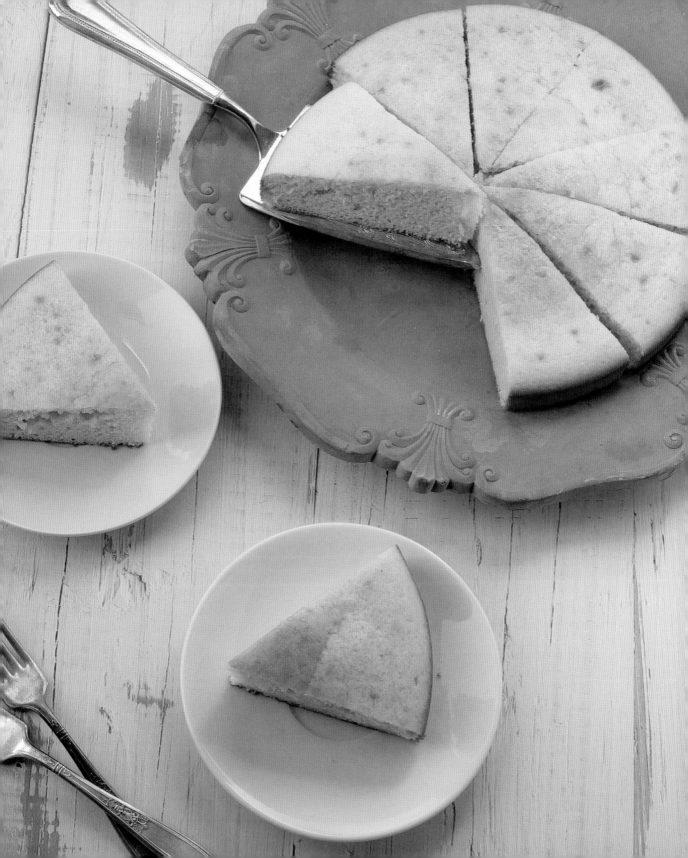

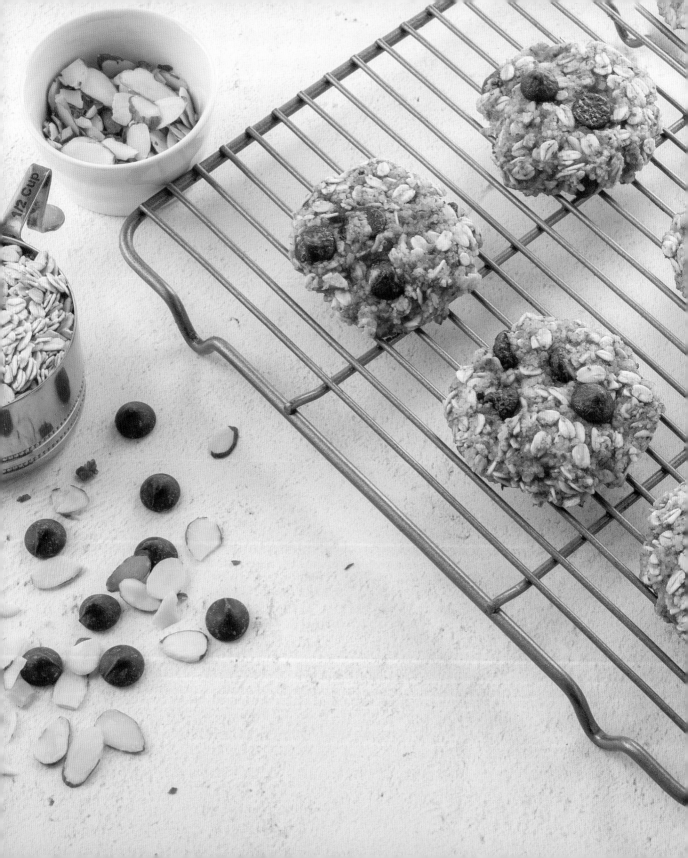

CHOCOLATE CHIP BANANA OAT COOKIES

MAKES 12 COOKIES

This is the perfect cross between an oatmeal cookie and a chocolate chip cookie. This recipe only has four ingredients and is so simple to make. Ripe bananas give the cookies texture and a natural sweetness, and the dark chocolate chips provide just the right amount of rich chocolate flavor. While sweets are encouraged in moderation on the Mediterranean diet, recipes like these cookies are a perfect addition because they use real ingredients and don't contain excess added sugars, butter, preservatives or artificial ingredients.

2 cups (286 g) raw almonds

2 medium ripe bananas

1½ cups (135 g) rolled oats

⅓ cup (55 g) dark chocolate chips

Preheat the oven to 350°F (175°C, or gas mark 4). Lightly spray a baking sheet with cooking oil.

In a food processor, pulse the almonds until they form a fine flour. Set it aside.

In a medium bowl, mash the bananas with a fork. Add the almond flour and the oats, and stir well to combine the mixture. Add the chocolate chips and mix to combine.

Using an ice cream scoop, form about 2 tablespoons (30 g) of the dough into a ball and then lightly press into a cookie shape. The cookies won't spread themselves, so form them into the size of a normal cookie.

Place the cookies on the prepared baking sheet and bake them in the oven for 7 to 9 minutes, until lightly browned. Allow the cookies to cool fully before enjoying.

TIP: These cookies only last about 2 days after baking, so freeze any extra in a container or freezer bag to last longer.

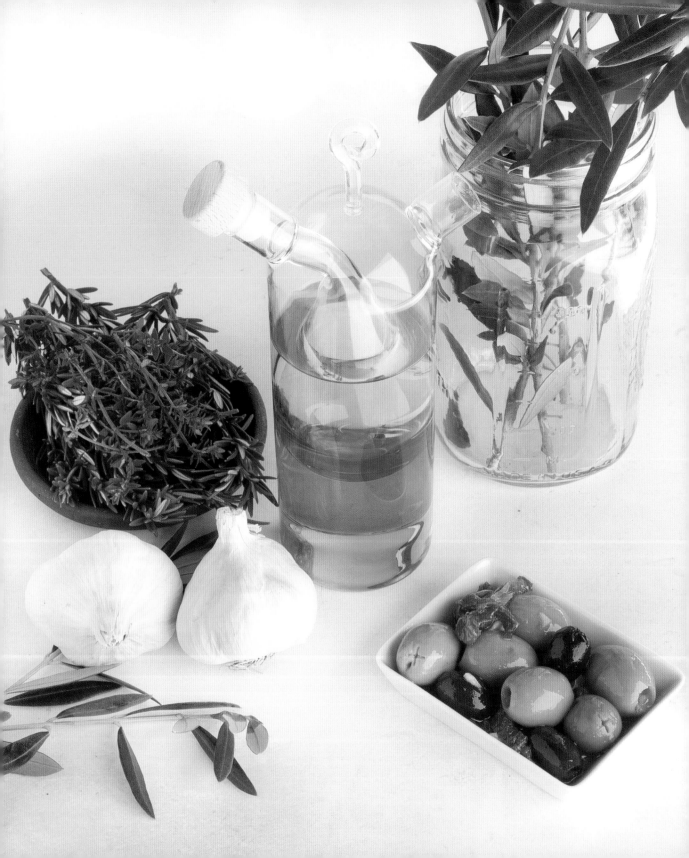

Timesaving SAUCES AND DRESSINGS

If there was one major takeaway from eating my way through France, Italy and Greece . . . it's that the key to many great dishes is the sauce. A plain bowl of angel hair pasta comes alive with a drizzle of olive oil, fresh garlic, a pinch of red pepper and freshly grated Parmesan. The fresh catch of the day gets elevated with a squeeze of lemon, some chopped herbs and capers. Even the simplest of ingredients can transform into a mouthwatering dish with the right sauce or dressing.

The Mediterranean diet emphasizes using ingredients such as fresh herbs, spices, fresh garlic, olive oil and citrus to season your food in place of excess salt, cream-based sauces or added fats. Experimenting with different herbs and spice combinations is a fun way to learn about flavor. Slowly stocking your pantry with dried herbs, an array of different spices, capers, garlic and flavored olive oils is a great way to set yourself up for fresh, flavorful meals.

This chapter contains some of my most-used and favorite ways to add flavor to dishes. Most of them can be made in advance, making them easy to prepare and have on hand in the fridge or pantry. A bowl of garden fresh tomatoes becomes an instant classic with a drizzle of Fresh Herb Oil (page 169), or a simple bowl of salad becomes a flavor explosion with a bit of Roasted Garlic Dressing (page 178). The Greek Seasoning Spice Blend (page 177) is always in my spice cabinet because it's a quick way to flavor everything from roasted vegetables to grilled fish.

TRADITIONAL TZATZIKI SAUCE *with* FRESH DILL

MAKES 3 CUPS (720 ML)

If I had to choose just one sauce to eat for the rest of my life, it would be this tzatziki. It's so creamy and it's packed with refreshing cucumber, dill and garlic. I use it on everything: as a dip for raw vegetables, on top of grilled chicken or as a spread on fresh Homemade Garlic and Herb Flatbread (page 45).

1 medium cucumber

3 cups (720 ml) plain Greek yogurt

3 cloves garlic, minced

1 tbsp (6 g) lemon zest

2 tbsp (30 ml) fresh lemon juice

1 tbsp (2 g) chopped fresh dill

½ tsp salt

¼ tsp pepper

Grate the cucumber and place it in a colander to drain. The key to thick and creamy tzatziki is to try and remove most of the water from the grated cucumber. You can also place the grated cucumber in a large paper towel and gently squeeze the water out.

Place the drained, grated cucumber in a medium bowl. Add the Greek yogurt, garlic, lemon zest and lemon juice. Stir well until all the ingredients are combined. Add the dill, salt and pepper. Stir again to combine.

Place the tzatziki sauce in the fridge for at least 30 minutes to allow it to re-thicken and the flavors to come together. The sauce can be stored in the fridge for 3 to 5 days; just stir it before serving.

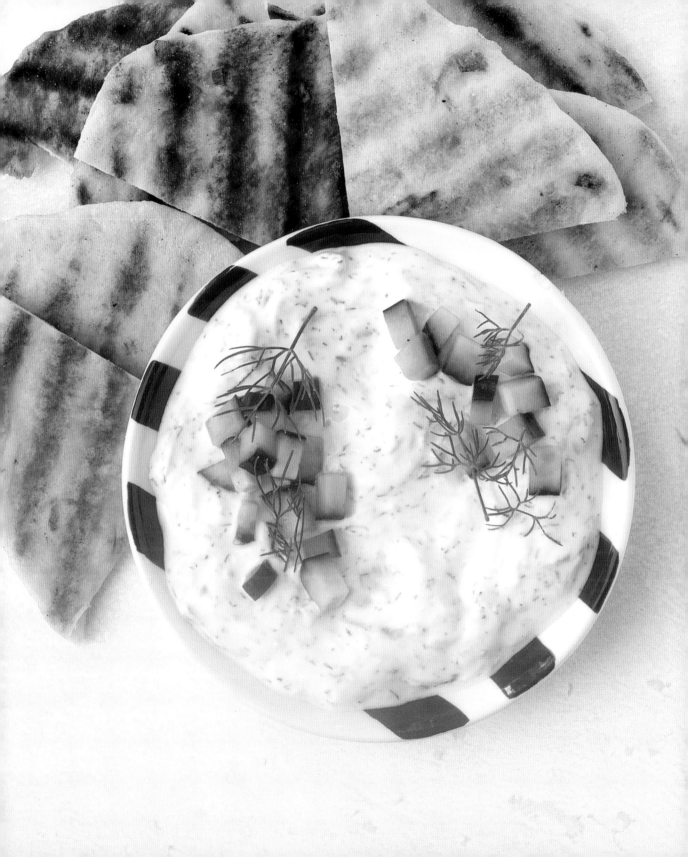

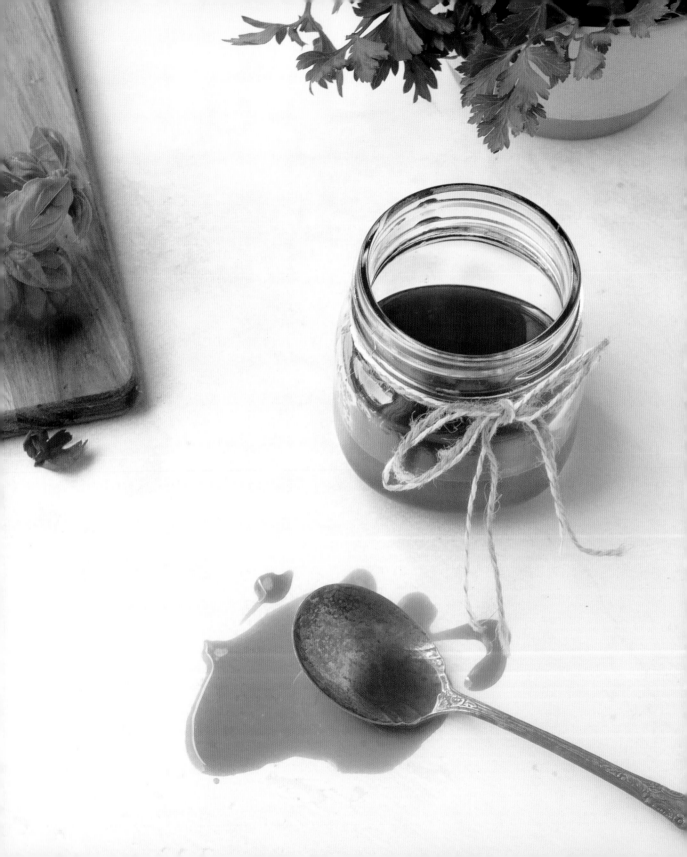

FRESH HERB OIL

MAKES 3 CUPS (720 ML)

Infused oil is a great way to use up fresh herbs. Use fresh herb oil as a dip for bread or drizzled on top of salads or sautéed vegetables. I also like it as a marinade for chicken or fish. It's so simple, but adds flavor to a dish that really brings it to life. You can use any soft herb such as basil, cilantro, parsley, tarragon, chives, etc. I prefer to remove the stems, but you can keep them on for additional flavor.

1 cup (200 g) fresh herbs, stems removed

2 cloves garlic, roughly chopped

¼ tsp salt

¼ tsp pepper

3 cups (720 ml) extra virgin olive oil

Start by blanching the fresh herbs so they retain their color when making the oil. Bring a large pot of water to a boil and add the fresh herbs, blanching only for 20 to 30 seconds. Remove with a slotted spoon and immediately add to the bowl full of ice water. After sitting in the ice bath for 30 seconds, remove and transfer to a paper towel–lined plate to drain.

Add the blanched herbs, garlic, salt, pepper and olive oil to a blender or food processor. Puree until thick and creamy, about 45 seconds. Pour the oil mixture into a food storage container and allow it to sit in the fridge for 24 hours. After 24 hours, strain it through a fine-mesh strainer. The oil is now ready to use. Store in an airtight container in the fridge; it will keep for approximately 4 days.

THE BEST HUMMUS *with* LEMON *and* ROASTED GARLIC

There are so many brands and flavors of store-bought hummus available, but nothing quite compares to the taste of homemade hummus. It's so creamy and smooth. You can also customize the hummus flavor by adding spinach, roasted bell peppers or fresh herbs.

1 head garlic

3 tbsp (45 ml) extra virgin olive oil, divided

1 (15.5-oz [439-g]) can chickpeas, drained and rinsed

½ tsp baking soda

3 tbsp (45 ml) fresh lemon juice

½ tsp salt

½ tsp ground cumin

½ cup (120 g) tahini paste

Paprika, for garnish (optional)

Start by positioning a rack at the top of the oven. Preheat the oven to 400°F (200°C, or gas mark 6).

While the oven is preheating, remove any loose outer layers from the garlic. Use a knife to cut off the top of the garlic—about a ¼-inch (6-mm) cut. Place the exposed head of garlic in the center of a large piece of aluminum foil, and drizzle with 1 tablespoon (15 ml) of olive oil. Wrap the garlic up in the foil so it's sealed tightly and place it directly on the top rack of your oven. Roast for 30 minutes.

While the garlic is roasting, place the chickpeas in a small saucepot and add the baking soda. Add just enough water so that all the chickpeas are covered, then bring the mixture to a boil over high heat. Continue to let the chickpeas boil for 15 minutes; if necessary, turn down the heat slightly to keep the mixture from boiling over. Remove the pot from the heat and drain the chickpeas into a fine-mesh strainer.

In a food processor or high-powered blender, add the chickpeas, lemon juice, salt and cumin. Remove your garlic from the foil and gently squeeze out the roasted cloves, they should come out very easily. Add all the roasted cloves to the food processor and puree everything together until well mixed. Add the tahini and puree the mixture together. Add 4 tablespoons (60 ml) of ice-cold water and puree until smooth and creamy.

Transfer the hummus to a serving bowl and drizzle with the remaining olive oil. Garnish with paprika for a pop of color, if desired.

TIP: Tahini is a paste made out of sesame seeds and can be found at most local and large chain grocery stores.

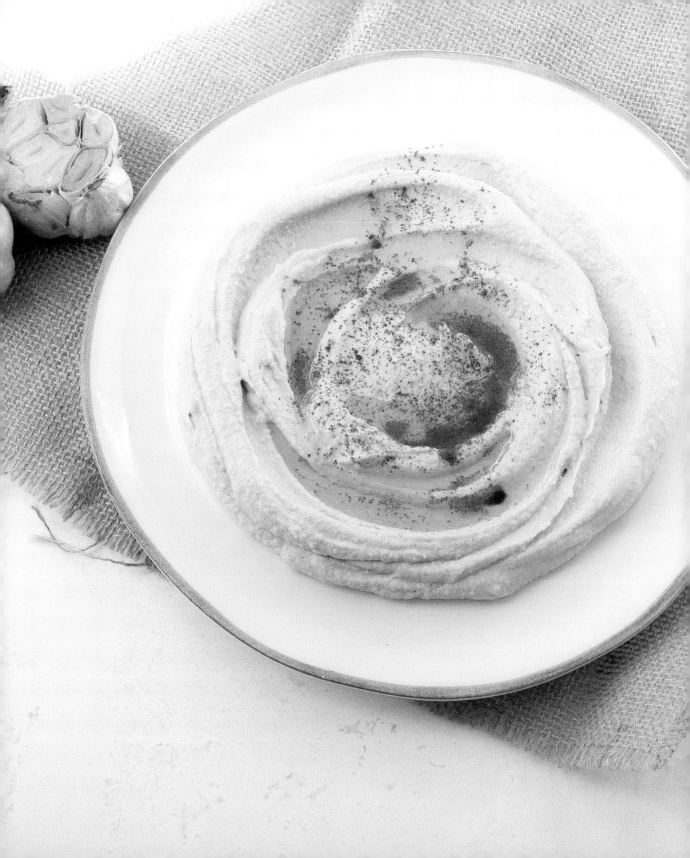

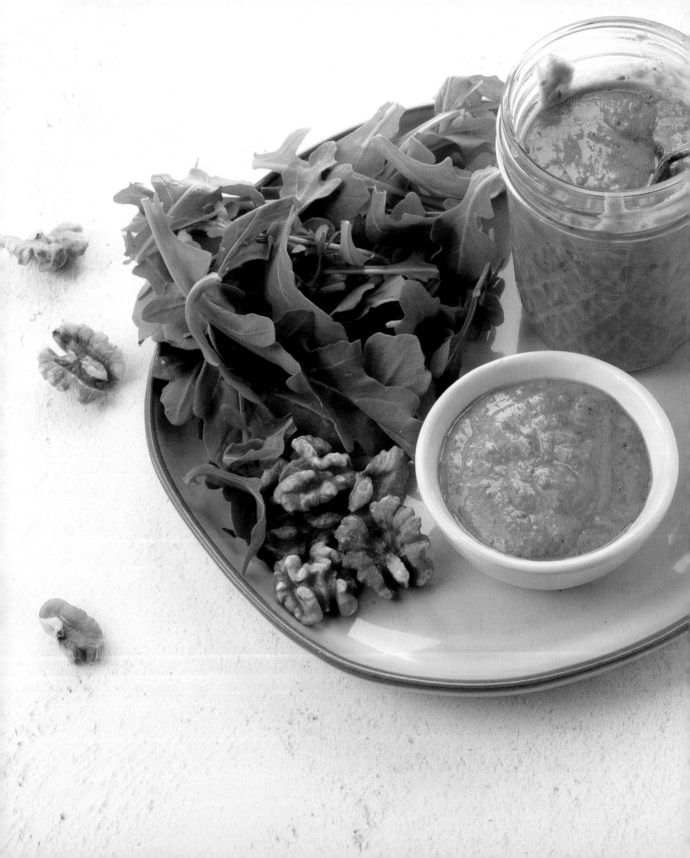

PEPPERY ARUGULA-WALNUT PESTO

MAKES 3 CUPS (680 G)

My love affair with pesto runs deep. It's so deep in fact that I planted three different basil plants in my garden last summer just because I could not stop making pesto. This recipe is a little more robust and peppery than the traditional variety because it uses walnuts and arugula instead of pine nuts and basil. It is also a good option when basil isn't in peak season.

To keep this recipe even more budget friendly, I recommend shopping for the walnuts in the bulk bin section of the grocery store, that way you can buy only the amount you need. I like having this on hand in the fridge to add to pasta dishes, grilled chicken, shrimp or even spread on top of a hard-boiled egg for a delicious midday snack. This pesto can be stored in the freezer for about 90 days: just drizzle a little olive oil over the top, cover it and freeze.

½ cup (59 g) walnuts

1 clove garlic

2 cups (68 g) arugula

1 cup (240 ml) extra virgin olive oil

½ cup (50 g) grated Parmesan cheese

½ tsp salt

In a food processor, combine the walnuts, garlic and arugula. Pulse until the mixture is finely chopped. While the food processor is running, slowly add the olive oil and continue to puree until well combined. Add the Parmesan cheese and salt, and pulse until well mixed.

TIP: You can store pesto in an ice cube tray in the freezer and then pop out individual frozen "cubes" of pesto as needed to toss into sauces or serve on top of pasta, grilled chicken or fish.

EXTRA CREAMY TAHINI DRESSING

MAKES 2 CUPS (480 ML)

There are a lot of recipes that just don't taste right without a creamy dressing or sauce. This dressing is my go-to when a recipe needs a little extra creamy texture. It's tangy and pairs perfectly with roasted vegetables or as a dressing on a simple salad.

½ cup (120 g) tahini paste

⅓ cup (80 ml) fresh lemon juice

1 tbsp (15 ml) extra virgin olive oil

3 cloves garlic, roughly chopped

2 tbsp (30 ml) apple cider vinegar

¼ tsp pepper

In a food processor, combine the tahini with ½ cup (120 ml) of hot water. Puree until the mixture is well combined and creamy in texture. Add the lemon juice, olive oil, garlic, apple cider vinegar and pepper. Puree everything together until well combined and creamy.

TIP: This dressing tastes great drizzled on top of roasted vegetables, like the Parmesan and Garlic Roasted Sweet Potatoes on page 147. I also love using it as a dip for raw veggies in place of ranch or cream-based dressings.

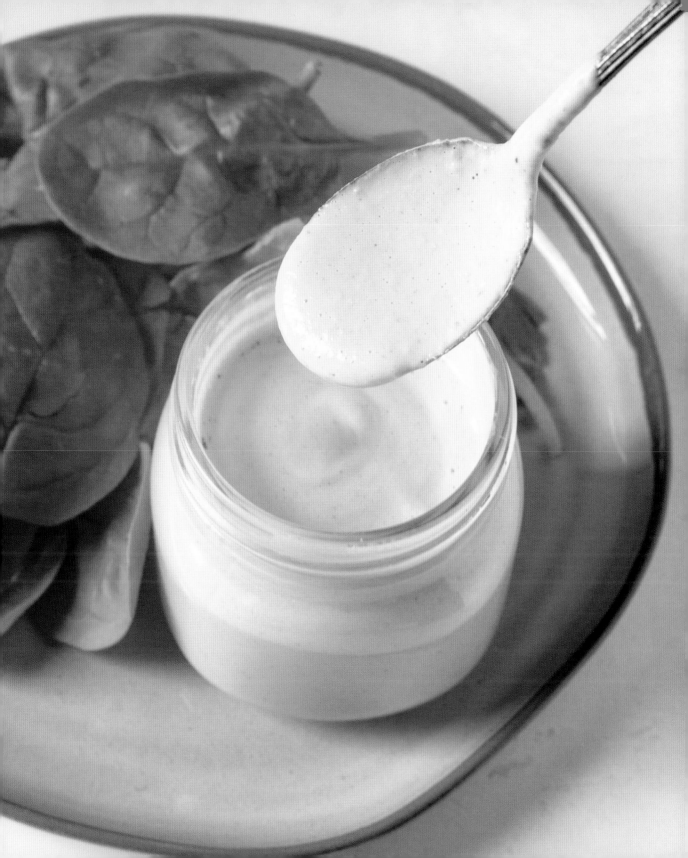

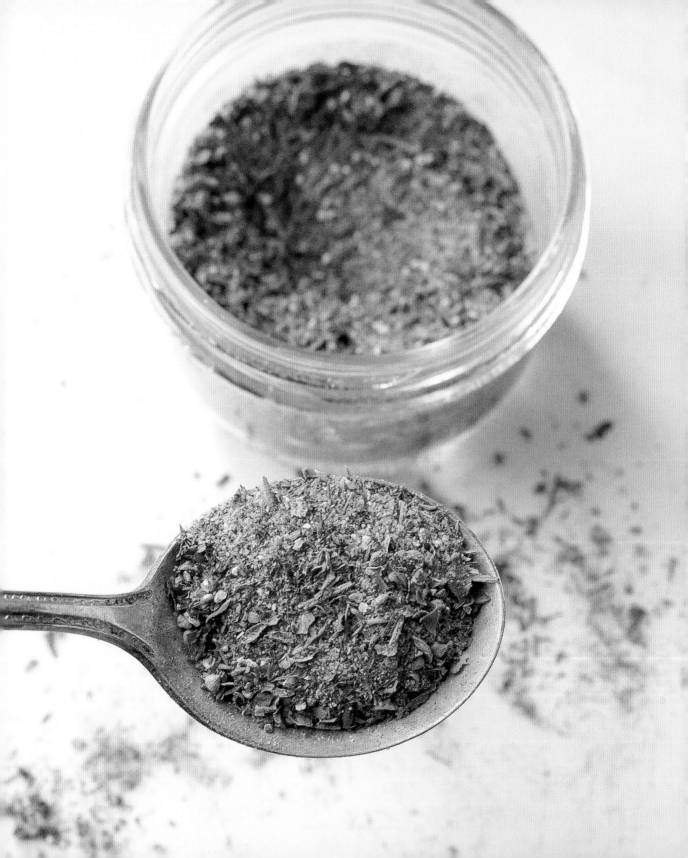

GREEK SEASONING SPICE BLEND

MAKES ½ CUP (53 G)

Taking just a few extra minutes to mix your own seasoning blend is a great way to create a spice you can keep on hand to make mealtime and cooking even easier. This blend is always in my spice cabinet, and I honestly use it at least twice a week. It makes a great addition to marinades, grilled meats and roasted vegetables. Mix it with olive oil to create amazing dressings and dipping sauces.

1 tbsp (5 g) dried basil

1 tbsp (1 g) dried dill

2 tbsp (17 g) garlic powder

1 tbsp (8 g) onion powder

2 tbsp (11 g) dried oregano

1 tbsp (3 g) dried rosemary

½ tbsp (2 g) dried thyme

½ tbsp (6 g) dried lemon peel

½ tsp ground cinnamon

½ tsp ground nutmeg

Combine the basil, dill, garlic powder, onion powder, oregano, rosemary, thyme, lemon peel, cinnamon and nutmeg in a glass jar or bowl. Mix until well combined. Store in an airtight container.

TIP: If you can't find dried lemon peel, you can substitute lemon pepper.

ROASTED GARLIC DRESSING

MAKES 1 CUP (240 ML)

If you've never had roasted garlic before, you are missing out on one of the best flavors available. And it's so simple with just a head of garlic and a bit of olive oil. This recipe uses that amazing roasted garlic flavor to create a thick, slightly sweet yet savory dressing that adds such a wonderful addition to salads, vegetables or even grilled meat.

1 head garlic

5 tbsp (75 ml) extra virgin olive oil, divided

2 tbsp (30 ml) red wine vinegar

1 tbsp (15 ml) lime juice

¼ tsp pepper

Start by positioning a rack at the top of the oven. Preheat the oven to 400°F (200°C, or gas mark 6).

To prepare the garlic for roasting, remove any loose pieces of the outer garlic skin. Use a knife to cut off a ¼-inch (6-mm) slice of the top of the garlic head. Place the exposed garlic head in the center of a piece of foil and drizzle with 1 tablespoon (15 ml) of olive oil. Wrap the foil up and around the garlic head so that it's sealed inside the foil. Place the foil-wrapped garlic directly on the top rack of the oven and roast for 30 to 40 minutes. Carefully remove it and allow it to cool.

In a food processor, add the roasted garlic by squeezing all of the roasted garlic out of the outer shell. Add the remaining olive oil, the red wine vinegar, lime juice and pepper to the food processor. Mix everything together until thick and creamy.

TIP: I often roast multiple heads of garlic at one time and store them in the freezer to pull out for later use.

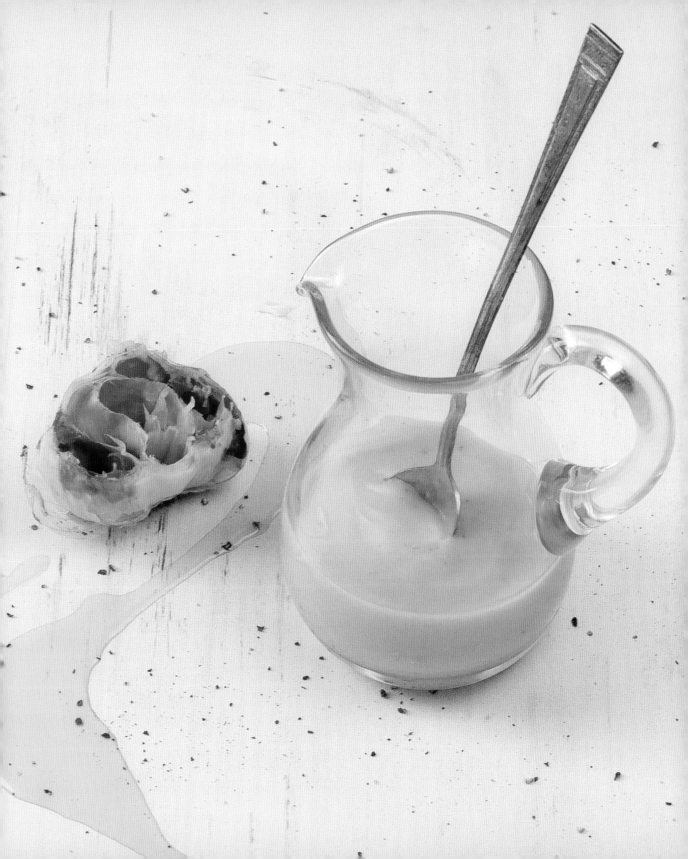

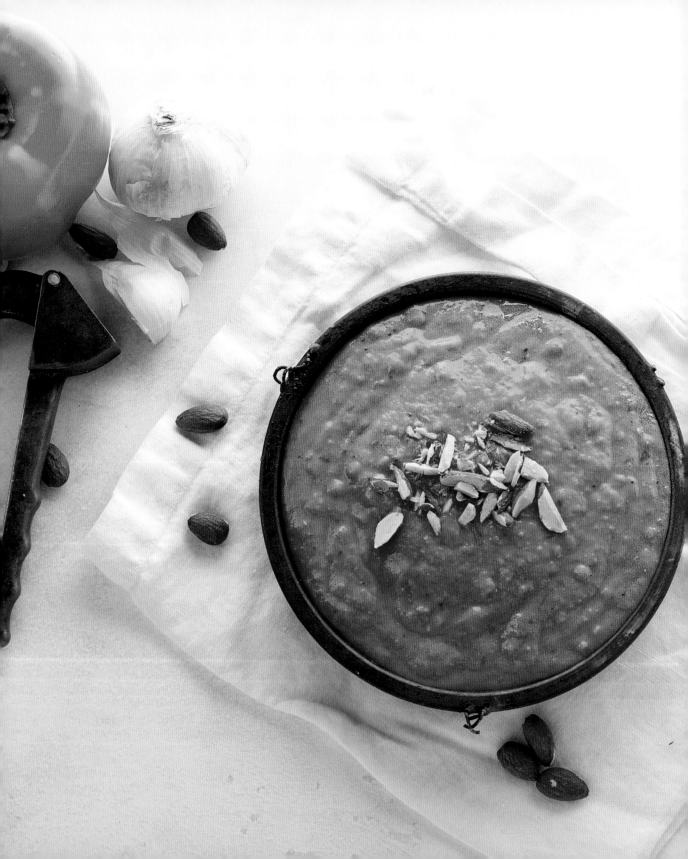

VIBRANT ROMESCO SAUCE

Makes 2 cups (480 ml)

This tomato-based sauce originated in Spain and it was intended to be eaten with fish. It is now a common sauce or dip served with meat, poultry and vegetables. The combination of ingredients creates such a vibrant and creamy sauce that adds so much flavor to a variety of dishes. I love making a double batch to have on hand in the fridge to liven up sandwiches, grilled chicken or even roasted vegetables.

1 (15.5-oz [493-g]) can roasted red peppers, drained

1 (14.4-oz [411-g]) can diced tomatoes with liquid

1 cup (143 g) raw almonds

¼ cup (15 g) chopped fresh Italian parsley

2 cloves garlic

2 tbsp (30 ml) extra virgin olive oil

1 tbsp (15 ml) fresh lemon juice

In a food processor, combine the roasted red peppers, tomatoes, almonds, parsley, garlic, olive oil and lemon juice. Puree until smooth and creamy.

TIP: You can kick up the heat on this romesco sauce recipe by using fire-roasted diced tomatoes and adding a pinch of red pepper flakes before pureeing.

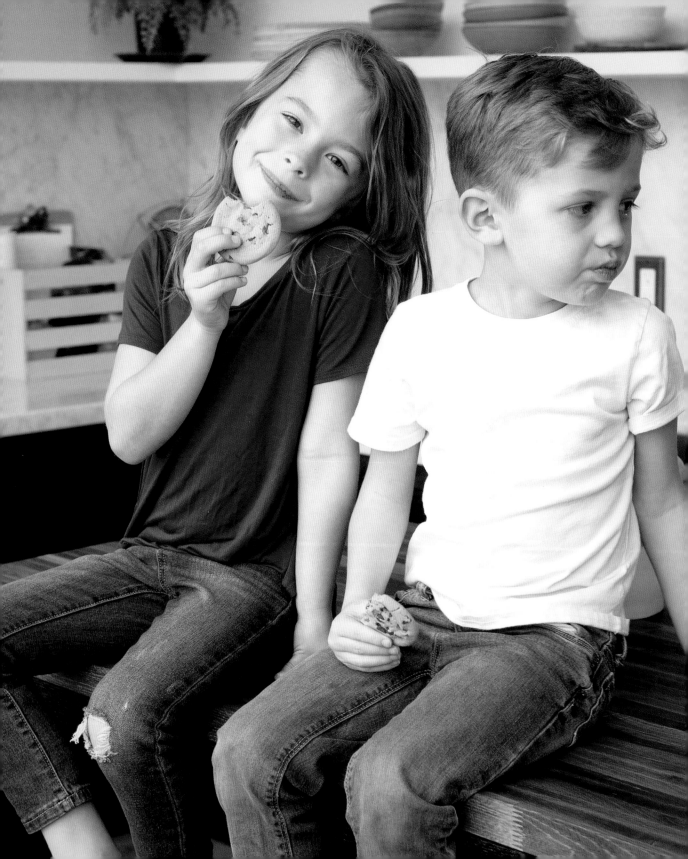

ACKNOWLEDGMENTS

Thank you from the bottom of my heart.

I honestly think I could fill an entire book up of just people that I want to thank. There are so many people that have, in some aspect of my life, led to this opportunity.

I'd like to start by thanking my family—Dan, Sophie and Race—thank you so much for always supporting me and pushing me to be better. Thank you for always being my recipe taste-testers and offering critiques and accolades with equal enthusiasm. Thank you for hanging in there with me through the writing process and for putting up with my long days and absent nights while I was cooking, photographing and typing away.

A huge thank-you to my friends and family who cheered me on during this entire process. Your support is never-ending and during the many, many times I didn't think that I could do it, your words and belief in me kept me going. Thank you to my mom and sisters for your help with the kids and your encouragement and feedback during this whole process. Thank you to my group of girlfriends who said they'll be the first in line to buy this book. I love you all.

Thank you to everyone who has ever visited, commented, shared or liked any blog post or social share from The Domestic Dietitian. I truly started out on a whim, thinking that maybe two people would ever read the blog (ahem Mom and Dan), but it's been so great to virtually connect with so many people and have your support. This little community brings me so much joy, and I hope that you'll continue to reach out.

And last but not least, thank you so much to Rebecca and the entire team at Page Street Publishing for taking a chance on me! Your expertise, patience and help through this whole process has been a dream.

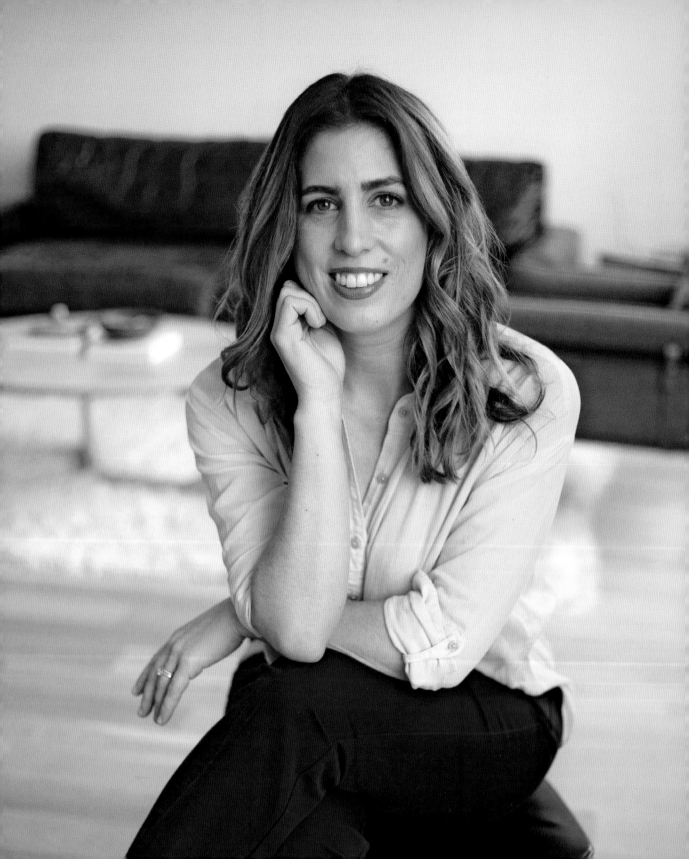

ABOUT THE AUTHOR

Brynn McDowell is a registered dietitian nutritionist with a bachelor's degree in nutrition and food science from San Jose State University in Northern California. After obtaining her registered dietitian credential in 2005, she went right to work providing nutrition support in a long-term care setting. Since then she's worked in food service, health care, nutrition counseling, management and consulting.

After the birth of her daughter in 2013, Brynn became a stay-at-home mom and started The Domestic Dietitian website as a way to continue to share her passion for nutrition while raising her family. She's continued to grow and expand The Domestic Dietitian as an authority on the Mediterranean diet by creating and sharing recipes, tips and health information designed to help others create a Mediterranean-inspired lifestyle in their own home.

In addition to being the sole creator of all content on The Domestic Dietitian, Brynn has contributed recipes for print in *Food & Nutrition* magazine and has contributed quotes and nutrition-related information for articles published online for Well+Good, PopSugar, *Reader's Digest*, *Men's Health*, Barefoot Blonde and *Shape*.

Brynn currently lives in Northern California with her husband, Dan, and their two children—Sophie (age 7) and Race (age 5).

INDEX